Menopause

Menopause

A Biocultural Perspective

LYNNETTE LEIDY SIEVERT

RUTGERS UNIVERSITY PRESS

NEW BRUNSWICK, NEW JERSEY, AND LONDON

LIBRARY OF CONGRESS CATALOGING-IN-PUBLICATION DATA

Sievert, Lynnette Leidy, 1960–
    Menopause : a biocultural perspective / Lynnette Leidy Sievert.
    p. cm.—(Studies in medical anthropology)
    Includes bibliographical references and index.
    ISBN-13: 978-0-8135-3855-6 (hardcover : alk. paper)
    ISBN-13: 978-0-8135-3856-3 (pbk. : alk. paper)
    1. Menopause. I. Title. II. Series: Studies in medical anthropology.
    RG186.S6664 2006
    618.1′75—dc22   2005028057

A British Cataloging-in-Publication record for this book is available
from the British Library.

Manufactured in the United States of America

In memory of
Marina Sánchez Conde de Paz

CONTENTS

FIGURES

TABLES

PREFACE

Women talk about the onset of menopause in various ways. Many cite the first time their menstrual period failed to make its regular appearance. Others describe the first time they threw off the blankets in the middle of the night. Some women complain of menstrual periods that flood more and more heavily each month; others encounter dusty, unused tampons in a bathroom cabinet. Although many women in the United States disdain the fuss made about menopause in the popular press, resent having to seek treatment for hot flashes, and dislike being reminded that the process of aging is marching forward, every woman who lives to sixty years of age with her uterus and ovaries intact is compelled, at one time or another, to say, "Oh, *this* must be menopause."

In general, ovarian biology is experienced as down there somewhere, internal, private, seemingly immutable. Women tell me that menopause is "out of our control," "natural," "biological." It is all of those things. Menopause—technically, the last menstrual period—is also a cultural phenomenon, "a time of despair," "a new phase of life." Culture, generally unacknowledged, alters the experience of menopause, the recognition of menopause, the timing of menopause, and the symptoms attributed to menopause. Culture is public, shared, and created. Culture is made visible in medical interventions, attitudes about aging, birth control policy, indications for hysterectomy, smoking practices, food resources, diet preferences, marital norms, breastfeeding customs, and timing of motherhood. All of these aspects of culture influence biology and contribute to variation in the age and individual experience of menopause.

The goal of this book is to tease apart culture from biology, although I would argue that it is impossible to think one can ever fully separate the influence of medicine, attitudes, diet, and health-related behaviors from any life change, menopause in particular. Cross-cultural comparisons facilitate the effort to separate the two; however, we find no simple dichotomy of cultural idiosyncrasies and biological universals. Some aspects of the biological process seem to be less plastic than others, less amenable to cultural influences. Nevertheless, in all settings and societies, culture and biology are deeply intertwined.

Biology and culture are enmeshed across the lifespan. Childbirth is an obvious example. The biology seems to be universally standard: an infant is pushed through a pelvic opening. But the biology of childbirth is not truly universal. Populations differ in the degree to which nutritional deficiencies and developmental difficulties are experienced by women during childhood. These early insults set the stage for later difficult or complicated childbirth in adult women (Merchant and Kurz 1993). Although the ease or difficulty of delivery is influenced by cultural interventions at the time of birth (Jordan 1993), culture does not interact with biology solely at the moment of study (at childbirth or at menopause); culture and biology are intertwined from conception to death.

Menopause is a rich topic of study. It occurs after forty to sixty years of living, that is, fifty or so years of eating, smoking, radiation exposure, sexual activity, pregnancies, weight gain, and maybe weight loss. Symptoms of menopause are complicated by climate, education levels, diet, weight, breastfeeding practices, smoking, alcohol intake, stress, and cultural expectations. The "treatment" of menopause is controversial. In fact, just trying to define menopause is a challenge, because menstruation may cease as a result of a hysterectomy, long before a woman runs out of viable eggs, while medically assisted pregnancy can extend the ability to give birth for years after menopause.

My own experience in the study of menopause spans two decades, from the beginning of graduate work at SUNY-Albany in 1986 to my current work with the anthropologists Daniel E. Brown and Lynn Morrison in Hilo, Hawaii; with Dr. Mario Carlos Gonzalez in Asunción, Paraguay; and with Dr. Jesus Zaraín García in Puebla, Mexico. Throughout these years and across six research sites, I have sought to understand age at menopause and symptoms associated with menopause as two aspects of human variation.

This text employs a biocultural perspective and a complementary lifespan approach. I explore evolutionary and cross-cultural understandings of menopause, as well as the influence of medicine. While the focus of biomedical research on menopause is too often limited to the effects of declining estrogen levels, many changes are concurrently taking place in women's lives as they age. The study of menopause presents tremendous opportunities for anthropologists and the holistic, comparative, and multidisciplinary strengths of the biocultural approach.

Three questions drive my interest in menopause: Why did menopause evolve? Why do some women experience menopause at forty-two, while others cycle like clockwork to the age of fifty-eight? Why does menopause pass unnoticed for some women, while others suffer from unrelenting hot flashes?

To set the stage for answering these questions, Chapter One reviews how menopause can be studied either as an event or as a process. Menopause is defined, and the biocultural perspective and lifespan approach are described. Chapter Two presents background endocrinology that serves as a reference for the remainder of the book. I discuss the ways in which human variation is divided into categories of normal and pathological and also examine hypotheses regarding the evolution of menopause and postreproductive life.

Chapter Three surveys past studies of menopause as well as the methodologies that are currently employed to measure symptom frequencies. Hysterectomies are discussed at the end of this chapter. Chapter Four also emphasizes methodology in explaining how age at menopause is computed for cross-population comparisons. In addition, I review the genetics of menopause and the factors associated with variation in age at menopause.

Chapters Five and Six focus on the symptoms associated with the menopause transition, with an emphasis on muscle-joint-bone pain/stiffness, depression, vaginal dryness and loss of sexual desire, and hot flashes. With regard to depression, I examine the history of involutional melancholy, particularly the evidence that dissociates depression from menopause. Chapter Six is devoted to hot flashes: the experience, the biology, their measurement, and factors associated with variation in hot flash frequencies within populations. Menopause as a result of chemotherapy is also discussed in this chapter.

Chapter Seven looks at a new phenomenon, the impermanence of menopause due to postmenopausal pregnancies and ovarian-grafting techniques. I conclude by noting future directions for research, including work on predicting age at menopause through imaging technology and the application of more consistent methodologies to achieve a better understanding of human variation in menopause across populations.

In Mexico there is a saying that "cada cabeza es un mundo," or each head is a world—each person creates or experiences a unique and separate reality. This saying describes what I've learned about menopause. Variation in the experience of menopause is related to many factors, including underlying biological variation, life experiences, health habits, and the influences of peers, family, physicians and other caregivers, and the media. At the level of the individual woman, every menopause is different.

This book, like my research, looks for answers to questions about menopause at the level of populations and species. *Menopause: A Biocultural Perspective* is written for students and researchers interested in the study of human variation, female fertility, biocultural and evolutionary frameworks, a lifespan perspective, and women's health. It is also written for women interested in understanding why certain changes occur during the transition from a reproductive to a postreproductive stage of life. When I started to study menopausal women, they were for me an exotic, anthropological "other." Now I have shared the lived experience of night sweats. To understand why they happen is helpful for all of us.

ACKNOWLEDGMENTS

The idea for this book originated with Catherine Panter-Brick. Alan Harwood nurtured the project, from start to finish, with tremendous patience and careful editing. Joan Merriman, Gillian Bentley, Julie Hemment, Elizabeth Krause, and Karen Mason improved an early draft. Two anonymous reviewers were generous in providing careful reviews that aided the entire manuscript. The manuscript became a book through the help, supervision, and editing of Adi Hovav, Beth Kressel, Marilyn Campbell, and, especially, Elizabeth Gilbert. For the uninterrupted opportunity to write in Hawaii, Japan, and Mexico, I am indebted to the hospitality of Greg Balogh and the Short-tailed Albatross Recovery Team, to Dan Brown, and to Lourdes Paz, Teresa Quintero, and Rosalia Escalera.

In choosing the topic of menopause, I am indebted to Patricia Draper for advising me, twenty years ago, to settle down and focus on something. I have been lucky to have encountered terrific mentors and colleagues from within the North American Menopause Society, from a menopause workshop in Madrid coordinated by Cristina Bernis Carro and Azucena Barroso, and from a menopause workshop in Beirut arranged by Carla Makhlouf Obermeyer. Robert Freedman and Janet Carpenter have been very generous colleagues. Over the years, I have also been encouraged and helped by Brooke Thomas, Barry Bogin, Gary James, Linda Gerber, Roberta Hall, Debra Anderson, Susan Goode-Null, and many other colleagues too numerous to name. I am especially indebted to Susan Hautaniemi Leonard.

For my work in Puebla, Mexico, I am indebted to Gustavo Barrientos, Clara Bowley, Regina Conceicao, Maribel Cuautle Cielo, María Graciela Espinosa Hernández, Jenny Foster, Charlene Franz, Zatcha Fuentes, Jesus Zaraín García, Gabriela Jiménez Zerón Sánchez, Olga Lazcano, Christopher Longcope, María Luisa Marván, Natalia López Montero, Kimberly Mueller, Lourdes Román, Ma. del Carmen Romano Soriano, and Yaratzet Specia Jiménez. That work was supported by a grant from the National Science Foundation (no. 9805299) and the Wenner-Gren Foundation for Anthropological Research. Matilde Espinosa Sánchez also contributed to my understanding of women's health in Mexico.

I learned how to study menopause in Greene County, New York, where 376 women were willing to talk to me, and I am indebted to Timothy Gage and others for their support. For my work in western Massachusetts I am indebted to Claire

Wendland, William Callahan, Susan Johnson, and Chris Canali. That work was supported by a Faculty Research Grant (1994) from the University of Massachusetts Amherst as well as the Wenner-Gren Foundation for Anthropological Research. For my work in the Selška Valley, Slovenia, I am indebted to Maruška Vidovič, Helena Horak, and Marge Abel. The project in Hilo, Hawaii, directed by Dan Brown, is ongoing. It has been wonderful to work with Dan, Lynn Morrison, Angela Reza, Harold Trefft, and UH-Hilo students. That work is funded by the NIH Minority Biomedical Research Support Program.

The work in Paraguay came about thanks to Ana Magdalena Hurtado, who introduced me to Mario Carlos González. Together we studied menopause among the Aché. With the help of Edith González de Troche, Mario and I learned about menopause among the Maká. For the work in Asunción, we are much indebted to the additional help of Maribel Gómez. That work was funded by a Faculty Research Grant (2003) from the University of Massachusetts-Amherst as well as a travel grant from the AAAS and the Women's International Science Collaboration Program.

Most of all, I am indebted to the women in upstate New York; western Massachusetts; Hilo, Hawaii; Puebla, Mexico; the Selška Valley, Slovenia; and various sites in Paraguay who graciously participated in the studies of menopause that form the foundation of this book. Finally, I am grateful for the unwavering support of Paul Sievert.

CHAPTER ONE

Introduction

Why study menopause? The answer is self-evident: because there are so many questions! Why do human females close down childbearing long before the end of life, while most chimpanzees reproduce until shortly before death? Why does menstruation end for some women at age forty-two, while others continue to menstruate at sixty? Why didn't my mother have any hot flashes, while other women remove strategic layers of clothing and visibly sweat?

Bring up the topic of menopause, and I'm more than happy to contribute curious observations, interesting hypotheses, and leaps of biological faith. Yet there are so many questions that I can't answer. Friends and colleagues at work ask, "I can't remember names anymore. Is that menopause?" "My left arm goes numb. Is that menopause?" "I want to have sex twice a day. Is that menopause?" "I'm more depressed than I have ever been. Is that menopause?"

Variation in age at menopause and in symptom experience *can* be understood at the level of the population by combining a familiarity with biology with observations of cultural difference. This book does present answers at the level of the population, but rarely about experience at the individual level. I have summarized much of what is known across a wide variety of populations, including those that are most familiar to me: upstate New York (where women talk about menopause as something natural, ordained by God), western Massachusetts (where women proactively smear themselves with yam cream and eat blue-green algae for menopausal health), Puebla, Mexico (where marital stress is a constant topic of concern among women of menopausal age), the Selška Valley, Slovenia (where menopause is an uncomfortable, taboo topic of conversation), and Asunción, Paraguay (where some women describe menopause as *un alivio*, a relief, but others volunteer the word *desesparación*, despair, as a menopausal symptom).

1

I focus on menopause both as a onetime event, the last menstrual period, and as an ongoing process, the transition from pre- to postreproductive life. These two points of view—event and process—reflect different approaches to the study of menopause, and both are necessary. I also examine the evolution and contemporary experience of menopause in a particular way—from a biocultural perspective.

Menopause as Event and Process

Menopause as an Event

Menopause is characteristic of human females, but very few other species experience a permanent cessation in the ability to reproduce followed by a long postreproductive life. Life history analysis allows anthropologists and biologists to compare traits across different species, such as rates of growth during childhood, age at sexual maturity, length of gestation (pregnancy), age at menopause, and maximum length of life. Mary Pavelka and Linda Fedigan (1999), for example, examined life history traits in free-ranging Japanese macaques (monkeys) to draw comparisons with human menopause. Japanese macaques are widely regarded as old when they reach twenty years of age, and only 8 percent of the studied population lived that long. Yet Pavelka and Fedigan found that most (81 percent) of the females that lived for twenty to twenty-five years were still reproductive. While all female monkeys ceased reproduction after twenty-five years, the end of their reproduction differed from human menopause in that the monkeys lived only an average of 2.1 years past giving birth for a final time.[1]

A twenty-five-year-old Japanese macaque is a very old monkey, showing advanced deterioration in all body systems. A fifty-year-old woman may feel the same way, but she is only at the midpoint of the human maximum lifespan. Menopause and postreproductive life are universal traits for human females who live through middle age, but only 3 percent of the macaques in Pavelka and Fedigan's study lived to age twenty-six (one year after their population wide termination of reproduction). Among macaques, menopause, if it happens at all, is an event that occurs very close to the end of life (see also Johnson and Kapsalis 1998; Takahata, Koyama, and Suzuki 1995).

In genetic terms, humans are more closely related to chimpanzees than to macaques. Do chimpanzees experience menopause? Graham (1979) studied thirty-five- to forty-eight-year-old captive chimpanzees *(Pan troglodytes)* and found that, although fertility declined after age thirty-five, most females were cycling regularly until death and all had at least one menstrual cycle within one year of death. Gould, Flint, and Graham (1981) showed that a forty-nine-year-old and a fifty-one-year-old chimpanzee demonstrated longer menstrual cycles, slightly different hormone levels (compared with those of younger chimpanzees), and reduced perineal swelling.[2] Although these two extremely old captive chimpanzees were showing perimenopausal changes, they were at the very end of their lifespans and had not stopped menstruating.

In a thirty-four-year study of wild chimpanzees in the Mahale Mountains of western Tanzania, Nishida et al. (2003) observed twenty-five females from middle age (18–33) until their death at age thirty or older. Postreproductive life was defined as the number of years between the birth of the last offspring and the year the female died, minus five years (because the average interbirth interval was sixty-six months for a daughter and seventy-two months for a son). Of the twenty-five females who died at age thirty or older (table IV, Nishida et al. 2003:114–115), fifteen were postreproductive—having no signs of pregnancy or estrus—for at least one year and six were postreproductive for five years or longer. Among the fifteen who were postreproductive for at least one year, the average age at death was 38.8 years. Among the six who were postreproductive for five years or longer, the average age of death was 40.2 years. It appears that chimpanzees, like macaques, can exhibit a short postreproductive life in the wild if they live long enough to be "old" (Nishida et al. 2003).

From a life history perspective, menopause is an event—a measurable trait—that can be compared across the macaque, the chimpanzee, and our own species, *Homo sapiens*. See figure 1.1, which compares data on various life events

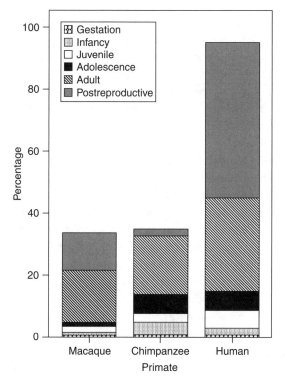

FIGURE 1.1   Life stages of the macaque, chimpanzee, and human.

Data drawn from Bogin (1999); Pavelka and Fedigan (1999); Dyke et al. (1986).

(length of gestation, infancy, childhood, adolescence, reproductive period, and post-reproductive period) across the three primates.

Menopause is also studied as an event by researchers interested in variation in the timing of the last menstrual period among human populations. In this case, investigators ask a sample of women their current age, the date of their last menstrual period, and—if they are not menstruating—whether or not they underwent a hysterectomy (to separate women with a natural menopause from women with a surgical menopause).[3] Information that may be related to the timing of menopause (for example, smoking habits) is also collected to understand variation in age at menopause within and between populations. This study of the timing of the last menstruation can be relatively rapid and straightforward, involving structured surveys and telephone, postal, or face-to-face interview techniques.

Menopause is also studied as an event within epidemiology—the study of patterns of disease. Epidemiologists consider the timing of the last menstrual period to be a risk factor (a measurable event) that helps to predict a woman's risk of breast cancer or osteoporosis. A late age at menopause is associated with a higher risk of breast cancer (Bulbrook 1991; Kelsey, Gammon, and John 1993; Sowers and La Pietra 1995). One hypothesis for this relationship, and for the increasing frequency of breast cancer in nations such as the United States and the Netherlands, is that women who experience more menstrual periods across the lifespan have greater exposure to monthly estrogen cycles. Estrogen stimulates breast tissue growth and with that growth comes a greater risk of genetic mutations that may result in an increased cancer risk. Consistent with this line of thinking, breast cancer risk is higher among women who have an early age at menarche (the first menstrual period—when estrogen levels rise) and among women who have a late age at menopause (when estrogen levels finally fall) (Eaton and Eaton 1999; Henderson et al. 1985; Pike et al. 1993).

In contrast to the relationship between age at menopause and risk of breast cancer, a late age at menopause lowers the risk of another disease of aging, osteoporosis, because estrogen helps to maintain bone density (Lindquist et al. 1983; Sowers and La Pietra 1995). At menopause, when estrogen levels fall, bone density drops dramatically. This drop in bone density has been used to market hormone replacement therapy (now called hormone therapy, or HT) (Brackett-Milburn, Parry, and Mauthner 2000; Palmlund 1997a; Worcester and Whatley 1992), because women who take estrogen (in pills or patches) after menopause experience significantly less bone loss. Yet one of the problems with HT is that, as just noted, exposure to estrogen increases the risk of breast cancer (Writing Group 2002).

Menopause is often treated as a onetime, life history event for cross-species and cross-cultural comparisons, as well as a medical event (a marker of estrogen decline). Women themselves, however, usually experience menopause as a more gradual, transitional process.

Menopause as a Process

The last menstrual period is an event that occurs within the transition from a reproductive to a postreproductive stage of life. In most countries this transition period is called the climacteric, but in the United States researchers speak more commonly of the "perimenopause" (Utian 1997). In general, the climacteric or perimenopausal transition begins when menstrual periods become irregular and ends one year after the last menstrual period. The word "climacteric" comes from the Latin word *climactericus,* meaning "of a dangerous period in life," or from the Greek word *klimakterikos,* from *klimakter,* meaning "a dangerous point, the rung of a ladder." "A dangerous period in life" may seem less favorable than "perimenopause"; however, because the word "climacteric" is used more often internationally, I employ both terms.

Marcha Flint, a biological anthropologist who studied menopause in India, Indonesia, and New Jersey, observed that menopause is related to the climacteric much as menarche is related to puberty (Flint 1975:161). In other words, menopause is the most prominent signal that the female body is exiting the reproductive period, just as menarche is the most prominent signal that the female body is entering it. There is a major difference, however, between menopause and menarche. While the first menstrual period is unmistakable, the last menstrual period is only certain in retrospect—enough time has to elapse before one can be sure.

To see how much time needs to pass for a woman to be sure she is past menopause, Patricia Kaufert, a Canadian sociologist, recorded the menstrual patterns of 324 women of menopausal age for three years (Kaufert, Gilbert, and Tate 1987). Every six months, women were interviewed by phone and categorized as menstruating regularly, having irregular menstruation, or not having menstruated for six months. Across the six interviews (three years), thirty-five women (11 percent) returned to regular or irregular menstruation after six months of amenorrhea (absence of menstruation). Relatedly, Phyllis Mansfield and colleagues (2003) used menstrual diary data from the longitudinal Midlife Women's Health Survey (now part of the Tremin Research Program, described in Chapter Three) to show that, during the five years preceding menopause, sixty-three women demonstrated ten distinct patterns of transition. Four of those women characterized their cycles as regular for a year or more, then changing for a year or more, then regular for a year or more, then changing again. Three women experienced twelve months of amenorrhea, only to have another period later on. This long period of unpredictability, waiting for that final menstruation, demonstrates why, cross-culturally, there are no rituals associated with menopause and why the clinical convention is for women to wait for at least twelve months before identifying their last menstrual period as the menopause event.

The increasing irregularity of menstrual periods is an external display of an internal process of hormonal change that precedes and continues throughout the menopause transition. Recently an over-the-counter, one-step urine test (Menocheck) was introduced by Synova Healthcare to detect elevated levels of follicle stimulating hormone (FSH), a physical concomitant of menopause. Two Menocheck tests taken five to seven days apart can determine whether or not FSH levels have increased and remained elevated. Menocheck was approved by the FDA (http://www.fda.gov/cdrh/oivd/homeuse-menopause.html) and may seem appealing from a commercial standpoint; however, a onetime test doesn't tell a woman very much during the process of the menopause transition. She could record an elevated FSH level one month, indicating menopause, and a low, normal FSH level the next. Just as her menstrual periods are irregular, her FSH levels are also up and down.

For example, in Malmö, Sweden, G. Rannevik and colleagues (1995) carried out a longitudinal, prospective study of hormonal change in 160 women for twelve years from pre- to postmenopause. They drew blood samples for hormone analysis every six months until one year after menopause and then once per year after that for up to seven years.[4] Because the study was longitudinal, investigators were able to look back and, at any particular point in time, know just how close a woman was to her last menstrual period. Table 1.1 shows the mean (average) serum levels of FSH from 84 months before menopause to 132 months after menopause along with the standard deviation (variation around the mean). Note how mean levels of FSH and the variation around the mean increase as menopause approaches.

Among women who were seventy-three to eighty-four months premenopausal, mean FSH levels were 2.6 ± 1.36 µg/l. In other words, all women had similar FSH levels, although some were closer to 1.0 (2.6 minus 1.36) and some were closer to 4.0 (2.6 plus 1.36).[5] Consider the standard variation for women who were one to six months premenopausal: 13.2 ± 7.5. In other words, while average FSH levels were about 13.0, some women were closer to 6.0 (13.2 minus 7.5) and others were closer to 21.0 (13.2 plus 7.5). All of these women were within six months of menopause. That is why a onetime test does not predict where any particular woman is in the course of her transition from pre- to postmenopause. With the assay used by Rannevik et al. (1995), a woman could have had an FSH level of 6 or 21 µg/l at the time of measurement and, either way, her menstrual periods stopped within the next six months. The physiological changes of menopause are best described as an up-and-down process, with enormous variation in FSH and other hormones. Month-to-month fluctuations are so great and so unpredictable that tests for hormone levels cannot determine just where a woman is on the path to menopause.

A process of hormonal changes underlies the symptoms[6] women associate with menopause. It follows, therefore, that investigators who study variation in symptom frequency study menopause as a transitional process, not a onetime event. Although menopause generally occurs between the ages of forty-five and

TABLE 1.1

Serum Levels of FSH

Months	N	Mean FSH μg/l	Standard Deviation
Premenopause			
73–84	31	2.6	1.36
61–72	49	2.8	1.98
49–60	75	3.8	1.91
37–48	94	5.2	3.55
31–36	107	5.3	4.66
25–30	127	6.5	5.34
19–24	136	7.9	5.90
13–18	146	9.3	6.54
7–12	152	11.1	7.47
1–6	154	13.2	7.50
Postmenopause			
1–6	146	18.5	6.47
7–12	119	18.2	6.21
13–24	158	18.7	6.46
25–36	157	20.3	5.67
37–48	156	20.5	5.61
49–60	151	19.5	5.78
61–72	147	19.7	5.64
73–84	136	19.1	5.22
85–96	115	18.9	5.29
97–108	89	18.5	4.90
109–120	65	17.8	4.48
121–132	51	16.6	3.80

Source: Rannevik et al. (1995).

fifty-five, premenopausal women aged thirty-five and older are sometimes studied in order to document the entire transition from regular menstruation to an absence of menstruation (Cramer and Xu 1996; Mitchell, Woods, and Mariella 2000). Often investigators ask open-ended questions to allow women to describe their own experience.

In Asunción, Paraguay, for example, in a study of age and symptoms at menopause, we asked, "In your opinion, what is menopause? What does it mean?" One quarter of the responses described menopause as a normal change that all women go through: "una etapa normal en la vida de una mujer" (a normal stage in a woman's life); "un proceso natural" (a natural process); "un ciclo por la cual la mujer pasa" (a cycle through which a woman passes); "un proceso de la vida" (one of life's processes); "es algo natural que hay que pasar" (it's something natural that one has to go through); "un período de cambios" (a period of changes). These answers give a sense of movement through time, menopause experienced as change across a temporal period rather than a one-time event.

Understanding menopause as a transitional process involves understanding the hormonal changes that accompany the transition, the symptoms associated with the process, as well as the various aspects of life that influence the experience along the way.

Defining Menopause

As defined by the World Health Organization, menopause is the permanent cessation of menstruation due to the loss of ovarian follicular activity (WHO 1981). This definition uses both a symptom that can be identified by a woman (the end of menstruation) and a sign that can be measured (the loss of follicular activity results in changes in levels of hormones). Investigators have generally agreed to define menopause as the last menstrual period followed by at least twelve months of amenorrhea (no menstrual bleeding). The advantage of this definition is that it identifies a single, measurable variable within the climacteric transition. This definition makes it possible to compute median or mean ages at menopause for inter- and intrapopulation comparisons. The definition also allows one to delineate a clinically normal range in age at menopause (for example, ages forty to sixty). Finally, this definition enables clinicians to identify women who are postmenopausal for medical "management." But while the last menstrual period is a clinically useful marker of an event, the average woman's sense of the process of the menopausal transition is better described by the term "perimenopause," a gray, difficult-to-define time period during which a woman wonders if each period of bleeding is the last.

Various staging systems have been proposed to differentiate premenopausal from perimenopausal and postmenopausal women (Mitchell, Woods, and Mariella 2000; Utian 2001) ranging from three to thirteen categories of menopausal status (for example, Oldenhave et al. 1993; Punyahotra, Dennerstein, and Lehert 1997). One set of criteria commonly used is shown in table 1.2. An advantage of these criteria is that only a few questions are required to differentiate among stages. For example, the investigator may ask: (1) Are you still menstruating? If the answer is

TABLE 1.2

Stages and Definitions of the Menopause Transition

Stage	Definition
Premenopause	Regular cycling. Having experienced a menstrual period during the two months prior to study.
Perimenopause	Irregular cycling. Having experienced a menstrual period from three to eleven months prior to study.
Postmenopause	Having experienced the last menstrual period at least twelve months prior to study.

no, is this because of pregnancy or lactation, hysterectomy (surgical menopause), chemotherapy (chemopause), or other medical treatment or condition? (2) When was your last menstrual period? If the answer is within the last two months, she is premenopausal. If the answer is within the last three to twelve months, she is perimenopausal (or amenorrheic for some other reason, such as pregnancy). If the answer is longer than twelve months before the interview, she is postmenopausal. (3) Are your cycles regular? If the answer is no, this helps to confirm that a woman is indeed perimenopausal. (4) Are you taking hormone therapy? Some women take cyclic HT that causes them to have periods. If this is the case, then it is difficult to determine if a woman is postmenopausal on the basis of the criteria in table 1.2.

The following data demonstrate how the criteria of table 1.2 can be applied with mixed success in studies of menopause. Among 755 women interviewed for a cross-sectional study of menopause in Puebla, Mexico, we found that 175 women had undergone a surgical menopause and 277 a natural menopause—defined as at least twelve months of amenorrhea. If perimenopause was defined as having menstruated within three to twelve months prior to interview, then only 9 women could be classified as perimenopausal. Another alternative was to group together all women who had menstruated within twelve months as premenopausal ($n = 303$), and this was done in the analyses (for example, Sievert and Espinosa-Hernandez 2003). This binary grouping is consistent with the WHO (1996) definition of premenopause, but by creating a "yes" or "no" scenario we lost the sense of menopause as a transitional process.

In Paraguay, we were more careful to ask about menstrual cycle changes, and 46 percent of the 234 menstruating women said that their menstruation had, indeed, changed in some way—heavier, lighter, closer together, or farther apart.[7] Twenty women could be classified as perimenopausal based on the criteria in table 1.2; they reported a last menstrual period from 61 to 240 days prior to interview. Of the 234 menstruating women (including the 20 who could be classified as perimenopausal), 77 women described their menstruation as "irregular." Of these, 14 said that their menstrual periods had become closer together and 63 said that their menstrual periods had become farther apart. Among those who said their menstrual periods were closer together, last menstrual periods ranged from 4 to 71 days prior to interview. Among those who said their menstrual periods were farther apart, last menstrual periods ranged from 1 to 240 days prior to interview. It quickly becomes clear that knowing the date of the last menstrual period doesn't necessarily tell the investigator whether a woman is perimenopausal. If a woman has a period every three months, but happens to menstruate the day before the interview, she will be identified by the generally accepted definition as premenopausal.

As discussed above, a onetime hormone measurement does not necessarily tell a woman whether she is pre-, peri-, or postmenopausal. Here we have confronted the difficulty of classifying a woman as pre- or perimenopausal solely on the basis of her menstrual cycle. Why is it all so complicated? Recall the WHO definition of menopause as the permanent cessation of menstruation due to the loss of ovarian follicular activity. To better understand what this "loss of ovarian follicular activity" looks like across the female lifespan, we have to begin with the female fetus.

In the human ovary (where female eggs are stored), approximately seven million oogonia are formed by the fifth month of fetal development. Oogonia are immature sex cells (eggs). Unlike males, female mammals (including humans) and birds do not continue to make thousands or millions of sex cells after an initial, early wave of production.[8]

The initial, exorbitantly high number of seven million oogonia declines to about two million oocytes in the ovaries at birth (T. G. Baker 1986) and 400,000 oocytes by the onset of puberty (Byskov 1978). Oocytes are almost fully developed sex cells (eggs). This drop in number of oocytes with age is a basic mammalian pattern, not unique to humans (Alcorn and Robinson 1983; T. G. Baker 1986; Nichols et al. 2005).

From puberty to menopause, monthly ovulation (when the egg is released from the ovary into the fallopian tube where it might be fertilized by a sperm) accounts for the loss of, at maximum, 400 oocytes. The vast majority of oocytes just simply degenerate, until comparatively few remain (Nelson and Felicio 1985; Novak 1970; Richardson, Senika, and Nelson 1987; Thomford, Jelorsek, and Mattison 1987). The degeneration of oocytes occurs through atresia, the process that involves the shrinking of either the oocyte itself or its surrounding follicle (Byskov 1978; Crisp 1992; Gougeon 1996; Guraya 1985). Because the oocyte and the follicle function as one developmental unit until the point of ovulation, terms such as oocyte loss and follicle loss are often used interchangeably. Figure 1.2 shows how follicles develop and grow within the ovary—from a primordial follicle (a few granulosa cells surrounding the oocyte) to a preovulatory follicle. Across the

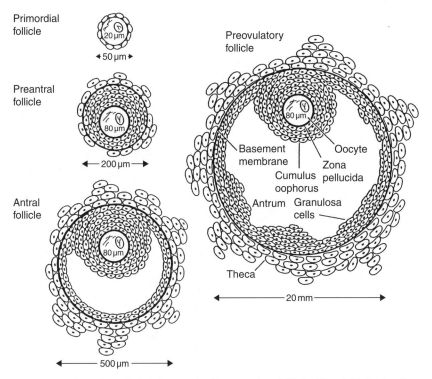

Primordial follicle

Preovulatory follicle

Preantral follicle

Antral follicle

Basement membrane
Oocyte
Zona pellucida
Cumulus oophorus
Antrum Granulosa cells
Theca

20 mm

500 μm

FIGURE 1.2 Growth and development of an ovarian follicle. The follicle develops from a primordial follicle, with only a few granulosa cells surrounding the oocyte, to a preovulatory follicle, with thick layers of granulosa and theca cells.

Figure p. 203, from *Clinical Gynecologic Endocrinology and Infertility*, 6th edition, by L. Speroff, R. H. Glass, and N. G. Kase, copyright © 1999 by Lippincott Williams and Wilkins.

lifespan, few primordial follicles will fully develop to a preovulatory follicle, compared with the hundreds of thousands of primordial, preantral, and antral follicles that will develop and then degenerate through the process of atresia.

At one time researchers generally agreed that oocyte depletion accelerated as menopause got closer. This belief was supported by data that, when graphed, showed a bend in the scatter of points representing numbers of follicles in relation to age (figure 1.3). This bend in the scatterplot was interpreted to mean a change in the rate of follicle loss around the age of thirty-eight or forty, consistent with the timing of the rise of FSH (Erickson 2000; Faddy et al. 1992; Gougeon et al. 1994; Richardson et al. 1987; WHO 1996). This interpretation made sense because, as its name implies, follicle stimulating hormone prompts more follicles to develop. The thinking was that increasing levels of FSH resulted in greater follicular development but, ultimately, a higher rate of follicle loss through atresia, because few developing follicles make it to the point of ovulation. The clinical

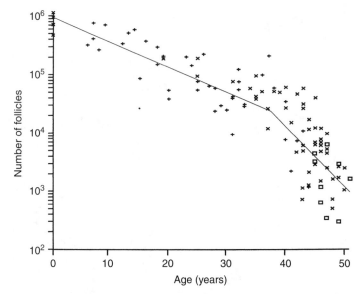

FIGURE 1.3 The most often cited model of follicular depletion, where follicular decay is exponential and the exponential rate changes abruptly at some critical age. Here the data from Block (1952, 1953) (represented by +), Gougeon, Ecochard, and Thalabard (1994) (represented by x), and Richardson, Senika, and Nelson (1987) (represented by blocks) have been redrawn on a log-linear scale (see Leidy, Godfrey, and Sutherland 1998).

Courtesy of Laurie Godfrey.

implication was that women should have children at younger ages because, physicians thought, the rate of follicle loss increased as menopause approached.[9]

This popular picture of follicle depletion (figure 1.3) has been misinterpreted.[10] The apparent bend in the rate of follicle loss was due to the log-transformation of follicle numbers (McDonough 1999). By converting numbers of follicles to a logarithmic scale on the y (vertical) axis, and by presenting age on a chronological scale on the x (horizontal) axis, the decline in numbers of follicles by age was bent so that it looked like the rate of follicle loss increased as women approached menopause. In fact, the number of follicles lost per unit of time is roughly constant during the years prior to menopause, an argument developed further in Leidy et al. (1998). Figure 1.3 continues to be widely used (for example, Wallace and Kelsey 2004); however, figure 1.4 shows the true decline in numbers of follicles across the lifespan.

With this correction in mind, we return to our explanation of the definition of menopause as the permanent cessation of menstruation due to the loss of ovarian follicular activity (WHO 1981, 1996). It has been hypothesized that when the number of ovarian follicles drops below a certain threshold, hormones such as estrogen produced by those follicles can no longer be secreted at levels high

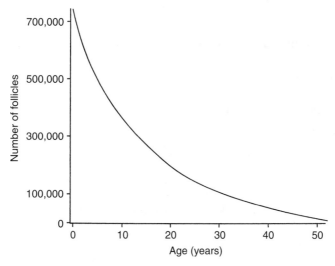

FIGURE 1.4 The shape of the true decline in numbers of ovarian follicles across the lifespan (see Leidy, Godfrey, and Sutherland 1998).

Courtesy of Laurie Godfrey.

enough to maintain menstrual cycles (Nelson and Felicio 1985; Wood 1994). This is the loss of follicular activity referred to in the WHO definition of menopause. This biological definition marks a measurable event that can be compared across cultures and plugged into models of disease risk.

There are, however, shortcomings to this definition. First, follicular activity can continue even in the absence of menstruation. For example, women who have undergone a hysterectomy (the removal of the uterus) may still have functioning ovaries. They may experience two kinds of menopause: first, the cessation of menstruation due to a hysterectomy, perhaps at age forty-two (no hot flashes), and second, the cessation of estrogen production due to the loss of ovarian follicular activity, perhaps at age fifty (and perhaps accompanied by hot flashes). Hot flashes are feelings of heat in the face, head, chest, or back of the neck that last about three to five minutes and are associated with the decline of estrogen. Second, follicular activity can end, but menstruation can continue through the use of cyclic HT. Women can experience periodic blood loss for decades beyond the loss of ovarian follicular activity by treating their hot flashes with a hormonal regimen that builds up the uterine lining, then allows the uterine lining to slough off (menstruation).

A third drawback to the WHO definition relates to how women experience menopause. Of the 470 women in Asunción, Paraguay, who were asked to define menopause in their own terms, although 31 percent of the responses defined menopause to be the end of menstruation, 13 percent defined menopause as the loss of the ability to have children ("termino del período reproductivo," the end

TABLE 1.3

Definitions Given for Menopause in Asunción, Paraguay

Definition of Menopause	Percentage
1. The end of menstruation	31
2. A normal life change	25
3. A negative life change	18
4. The end of fertility	13
5. Don't know	8
6. Other (e.g., beginning of old age, end of desire for sex)	5

Source: Unpublished data.

Note: Some women gave more than one definition, for a total of 501 responses.

of the reproductive period; "perdida de la capacidad de tener hijos," the loss of the ability to have children). See table 1.3.

The WHO definition does not address this perception that menopause is equivalent to the loss of reproductive ability, because biological evidence supports a separation between the loss of fertility and the end of menstruation. Fertility (giving birth to offspring) ends well before the end of menstruation, as demonstrated in studies of women receiving sperm donation (Federation CECOS, Schwartz, and Maynaux 1982; van Noord-Zaadstra et al. 1991) and oocyte donation (Abdalla et al. 1990). Older women have more difficulty getting pregnant because they have fewer healthy eggs. In addition, both historical and cross-cultural evidence have demonstrated that, at the population level, the end to female fecundity (the ability to become pregnant and/or to maintain a pregnancy) ends an average of five to ten years prior to the end of menstruation (Gage et al. 1989; Wood 1994). For most women, fecundity declines around the early to midforties.

That said, women still perceive menopause to be a marker for the end of childbearing because most women have no other "window" into the state of their ability to conceive. The end of menstruation can, therefore, be an emotion-laden event. Some women react to the cessation of menstruation with relief (no more birth control); others describe deep sadness because they can no longer bear children. A woman in western Massachusetts explained to me, "I could have had twenty children. I loved having children." How many did you have? "Seven. But it was so easy then. I could fill a grocery cart for forty dollars. I wish I could have had more children."

In Asunción, some women described the loss of fertility in positive terms, such as "Un alivio para las mujeres. No preocuparse por la menstruación y embarazo" (Relief for women. No worry about menstruation and pregnancies). Others had mixed feelings as they described "el final de una etapa de reprodución" (the end of a stage of reproduction); "incapacidad de tener hijos" (inability to have children); "la culminación del período fertil" (the culmination of the fertile period). Explained one woman when asked to define menopause, "Ya no se puede tener hijos" (One can no longer have children).

If the cessation of menstruation signifies, as it does for many women, the end of fertility, then could tubal ligation (having one's "tubes tied")—a medical procedure that ends fertility—be considered a "cultural" menopause? No, because sterilization does not bring about the end of menstruation. From a different perspective, if medically assisted postmenopausal pregnancies can extend the ability to give birth for ten or fifteen years beyond the cessation of menses, then what does menopause mean? Simply: the end of menstruation.

The Biocultural Perspective

This text utilizes a biocultural perspective, which offers a "comprehensive view of humans" (McElroy 1990:244) by showing that biology and culture are intertwined in "a continuous feedback relationship of ongoing exchange" (Lock 1998:410). Biological variables are both cause and effect (Wiley 1992). Evolution shapes the biological constraints, for example in the timing of menopause (Peccei 1995). In addition, the biocultural perspective examines the developmental and environmental processes that bring about human variation (Bogin 1999; Worthman 1993), for example, in menopausal symptoms.

Biology and culture can be brought together into a comprehensive study of humans in myriad ways. The holism of the biocultural framework allows anthropologists to explore a wide range of research topics, across any length of time, using different measures of fitness (for example, reproductive success or rate of childhood growth) to understand how biology, culture, and the environment interact to shape a particular phenomenon.

Some anthropologists ask questions on an evolutionary scale, hundreds of thousands or millions of years in length. These questions are often about macroevolution—the formation of new species through the accumulation of evolutionary changes produced across many generations. In our own evolutionary history, earlier species evolved into later species; for example, *Homo erectus* (a species active at least 1.8 million years ago) was ancestral to our own (very recent—perhaps only 150,000 years old) species of *Homo sapiens*.

In terms of the biocultural perspective, paleoanthropologists are interested in how and why brain size and complexity increased throughout our evolutionary history from a cranial capacity and surface morphology (size and shape) similar to that of a chimpanzee (about 400 cm³) to our present highly convoluted brain surface and large brain size (about 1,400 cm³). Those with a biocultural orientation propose a feedback loop between cognition and tool manufacture. Increasing cranial capacity and structural complexity may have been associated with increasing cognitive skills—including social and language skills (Falk 1992)—that influenced, and in turn were influenced by, the development of more sophisticated tools (Wynn 2002).

The mechanism explaining the changing brain size across time is natural selection. Technologically and socially skilled hominids would have had differential access to food and mates. According to Dean Falk (1992), a paleoneurologist, "hominids who (a) stayed alive, and (b) bred successfully would have been targets of natural selection. Presumably, many aspects of intelligence would have facilitated such selection" (178) resulting in increasing cognitive skills over thousands of years and expanding brain capacity. The interaction of behavior (tool manufacture) and biology (brain size and complexity) through evolutionary time illustrates the biocultural approach.

Macroevolution results in new species, but all evolutionary changes are ultimately the result of microevolution—changes in allele frequencies within a population from generation to generation. (Alleles are different versions of the same gene, such as the A, B, and O alleles for blood type.) The mechanisms underlying these changes are the forces of evolution. One of those forces is natural selection. For natural selection to work, first, there must be variation among individuals who have a particular trait within a population (such as age at menopause). Some aspect of variation will be advantageous within a particular context and the individuals with those beneficial traits will be selected for. "Selected for" means that they will (a) stay alive and (b) produce more offspring compared with individuals with slightly different traits.

Sometimes human biologists interested in contemporary populations also incorporate an evolutionary perspective. For example, Katherine Dettwyler (1995a) argues that to investigate breastfeeding as a biocultural phenomenon, we must begin with an understanding of "our evolutionary inheritance" (39) as vertebrates, mammals, and primates (figure 1.5). Humans are shaped by "the hominid blueprint" (39) that developed during our own particular evolutionary path. Because we are mammals, humans produce milk from mammary glands; however, human milk is different from the milk of other mammals because it evolved through natural selection to meet the specific nutritional and immunological needs of human infants. Once we understand our evolutionary inheritance (biology), we can better investigate breastfeeding as a heavily "culturalized" activity (Dettwyler 1995a:41).

Similar in evolutionary scope is Margie Profet's (1992) proposal that morning sickness evolved through natural selection as an adaptation to the ingestion of plant toxins during the PlioPleistocene epochs (five million to ten thousand

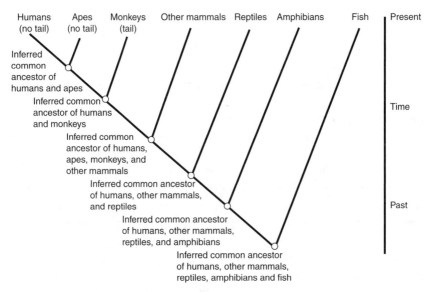

FIGURE 1.5 Evolutionary relationships among humans, apes, monkeys, other mammals, reptiles, amphibians, and fish.

Redrawn from Relethford (2005:225).

years before the present), when our hominid ancestors lived in small, mobile communities with access to a wide variety of plant foods and some lean meats (Eaton, Eaton, and Konner 1999). In Profet's scenario, women who avoided (or vomited) plant substances that could harm a developing embryo enjoyed greater reproductive success and had more children. Others have hypothesized that morning sickness evolved to avoid not plant toxins but parasites and pathogens in meat (Flaxman and Sherman 2000). In either case, there is thought to be a biocultural relationship within our evolutionary history between subsistence patterns such as hunting and gathering (culture) and morning sickness (biology). This interest in the "environment of evolutionary adaptedness"—the context within which our ancestors evolved (Hrdy 1999)—is shared by many anthropologists, including those who study menopause within contemporary populations (Hawkes, O'Connell, and Blurton Jones 1997).

Some anthropologists apply an adaptationist perspective to understand how social behavior benefits contemporary individuals by increasing or decreasing fertility. These anthropologists study the interaction of biology and culture among contemporary peoples—hunters and gatherers, pastoralists, agro-pastoralists, and agriculturalists (for example, Bentley, Paine, and Boldsen 2001; Ellison 2001a,b; Hawkes, O'Connell, and Blurton Jones 2001; Hill and Hurtado 1996; Kaplan et al. 2000; Panter-Brick 2002)—within a variety of ecological conditions.

For example, Gibson and Mace (2002) studied women in southern Ethiopia to understand the effects of labor-saving technology (a recent water-supply project) on women's "energy budgets." They predicted that energy formerly used by women in making long trips for water (up to six hours per day, for up to thirty kilometers, to carry loads of twenty to twenty-five liters) would now be diverted into reproductive effort. Eventually, this would increase fertility. Villages with and without water taps were compared to show that access to water taps (culture) was, indeed, associated with an earlier return to menstruation and pregnancy (biology) after giving birth.

The questions formulated from an adaptationist perspective are driven by hypotheses derived from the theory of natural selection. In keeping with natural selection, the measure of fitness is fertility—in evolutionary terms, those who leave more offspring are more successful. As demonstrated above, fertility varies in relation to energy expenditure. Fertility is also associated with other aspects of culture, such as marriage patterns (including age at marriage, or polygyny versus monogamy), religion, and differential access to nutritional resources. With regard to menopause, an adaptationist perspective allows evolutionary ecologists to investigate how grandmothering—a behavior that differs from culture to culture— may have resulted in the evolution of a long postreproductive life. If postreproductive, hominid grandmothers could provide care for their grandchildren (Hawkes, O'Connell, and Blurton Jones 1997), and if this investment resulted in the survival of more grandchildren, then, the argument goes, menopause followed by a long postreproductive life would have been selected for as favorable traits.

The biocultural perspective is also applied by human biologists who use an ecological model to study contemporary populations. These studies expand the definition of "fitness" beyond fertility and mortality. In other words, in addition to testing whether or not particular individuals (a) stay alive and (b) produce more offspring, the ecological model also includes other measures of fitness, such as growth (distance and velocity, or how much and how fast), work capacity, blood pressure, morbidity (disease or sickness), and other measures of the quality of life. Their questions focus on explaining human variation through genetic, developmental, and nongenetic physiological change (P. T. Baker 1984; McElroy and Townsend 2004; Moore et al. 1980; Thomas, Gage, and Little 1989; Wiley 2004). For example, Ivy Pike (1999) has studied how seasonal differences (wet season/dry season) influence food availability, workloads, and exposure to pathogens. She investigated whether seasonality influenced weight gain among pregnant Turkana women in Kenya.

The ecological model is a holistic paradigm that examines the relationships among biology, culture, and the environment with an emphasis on human adaptation (D. E. Brown 1981; Frisancho 1993; Gonzalez Quintero and Lopez Alonso 2003; Kormondy and Brown 1998; Wiley 2004). Figure 1.6 shows one conceptualization of these interactions.

A classic example of the biocultural model applied at the level of the population is the effect of dairying, a cultural practice, on human biology. All mammals

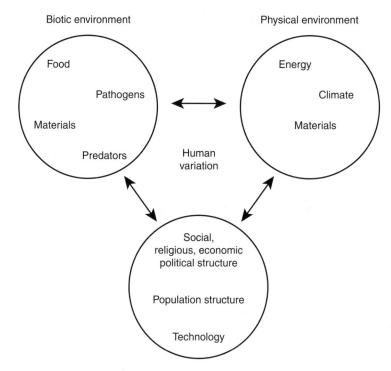

Biotic environment

Physical environment

Food

Pathogens

Materials

Predators

Energy

Climate

Materials

Human
variation

Social,
religious, economic
political structure

Population structure

Technology

Cultural-demographic environment

FIGURE 1.6 A biocultural model for examining human variation.

Figure 15.1, from *Human Population Biology: A Transdisciplinary Science*, edited by
Michael A. Little and Jere D. Haas, copyright © 1989 by Oxford University Press,
Inc. Used by permission of Oxford University Press, Inc.

produce milk, but the ability to digest this milk is not lifelong. Instead, the ability
to digest lactose, the milk sugar, declines as infancy ends (Durham 1991). Some
human populations retain the ability to digest lactose; a high degree of lactose
tolerance (the ability to digest milk) is found in populations of people with ancestral ties to northern Europe or western Africa, where dairying has been practiced
for thousands of years (Simoons 1978). There was a selection for lactose tolerance
in those populations, probably through a higher level of fertility associated with
the ability to digest milk, because milk provided new sources of nutrients, especially calcium, vitamin D_3, protein, and fats (Bogin 1998). This is a remarkable
example of how culture can influence microevolution. A change in allele (gene)
frequencies made it possible for particular populations to digest milk.

While the evolution of lactose tolerance is an excellent illustration of the
role of natural selection in human adaptation, scientists using an ecological
model are not always explicit about the evolutionary theory underlying their
work. Often this is because the trait of interest (such as hot flashes) has no clear

adaptive advantage, but is an aspect of human variation that demonstrates ways in which culture, biology, and the environment interact. Rather than explaining how a particular trait is adaptive (and selected for by natural selection), biocultural researchers frequently find that it is human plasticity that has evolved through natural selection, allowing for changes in a particular trait across space and time in relation to particular stressors.

For example, age at menarche is a sensitive measure of population health, because the average age at menarche changes in response to nutritional excess or deficits (Bogin 1999; Eveleth and Tanner 1990). A dramatic example is the way in which age at menarche varies across birth cohorts before and after a war (Prebeg and Bralic 2000; van Noord and Kaaks 1991). For example, among girls in the city of Šibenik, Croatia, mean age at menarche had been decreasing since World War II, consistent with a secular trend in age at menarche that occurred across the globe during the twentieth century. War came to Šibenik in September of 1991, and attacks lasted through August of 1995. Prebeg and Bralic (2000) showed that mean age at menarche reversed its downward secular trend and rose from 12.9 years in 1985 to 13.1 years in 1996. Girls who lost a family member during the war experienced menarche at a still older mean age of 13.8 years. The physiological capacity to shift age at menarche earlier or later, in response to environments that help or hinder reproduction, was selected for over millions of years of hominid evolution.

Some biocultural researchers focus on social and psychological factors associated with stress and disease outcomes, such as depression or hypertension. Behavioral factors (for example, smoking or poor diet) may increase an individual's risk of disease. From a biocultural perspective, other, less measurable factors are also associated with the development of these diseases, including a person's social circumstances, beliefs, and attitudes. William W. Dressler, a leader in this area of study, argues that the central problem in cross-cultural studies of stress is that the factors that cause stress and the factors that reduce stress are culture specific (Dressler 1996). They are not just items on a checklist that can be ticked off and compared; the researcher must situate the factors at a local level. Thus Dressler (1996) borrows Clifford Geertz's term "local knowledge" to talk about culture as meanings that define appropriate behaviors and organize human relationships. Similarly, "local biology" refers to the ways in which physiological processes shape and are shaped by the sociocultural milieu in which they are embedded (Hinton 1999; Kleinman 1995; Lock 1993; Melby, Lock, and Kaufert 2005; Worthman 1993, 1999; Worthman and Kohrt 2005).

In multiple research settings, Dressler investigated the effects of "lifestyle incongruity"—defined as the degree to which lifestyle (including characteristics such as items owned and adoption of "cosmopolitan" behaviors) exceeds the typical characteristics of one's occupational class—on blood pressure, depressive symptoms, and serum lipids. Measures of lifestyle and occupational class are variables that must be understood in relation to cultural context. Dressler found that within the cultures of St. Lucia, Brazil, Mexico, and Alabama, people with greater lifestyle incongruity demonstrated higher blood pressure (reviewed in Dressler 1995, 1996). Dressler and his colleagues have also contributed to an understanding of health in relation to "cultural consonance"—a measure of how closely an individual's behavior approximates the "guiding sensibilities" of his or her own culture—through studies of blood pressure in relation to lifestyle and social support norms (Dressler and Bindon 2000:246).

Other researchers have also focused on cultural variables such as social support or "social power" in relation to physiological outcomes. Social power— defined as the perceived potential to influence outcomes—is achieved through interactions with others. Increasing social power reduces stress within local contexts. For example, among the Fulbe of Mali in West Africa, Dominique Simon and colleagues investigated social power through such questions as whether a woman would return to the market to ask for her money back when she discovered she had been short-changed. They found that women who scored higher in terms of passivity/helplessness were more likely to have children who were malnourished. A child's nutritional status was also associated with seasonality, maternal age, and whether the mother had a Koranic education typical of the area (Simon, Adams, Madhavan 2002). The ecological model is holistic, encompassing social support, attitudes, subsistence strategies, diet, seasonality, and war with an interest in a variety of outcomes, including growth, weight gain, blood pressure, and any number of other measures of the quality of life.

A final way in which a biocultural approach is understood is by anthropologists who emphasize political-economic relationships and their effect on human biology (Goodman and Leatherman 1998; Leatherman and Goodman 1997; Smith and Thomas 1998). Within this approach, economic and political processes lead to specific patterns of biological stress and compromised biologies further threaten the integrity of social processes.[11]

For example, according to Bogin and Loucky (1997), short height can be an indicator of physical, economic, or political stress. They showed how the children of Maya immigrants born in the United States grew an average of 5.5 cm taller than their age mates living in Guatemala. They argued that migration to the United States breaks the cycle of poverty into which most Guatemalan Maya are born and that plasticity in the growth of Maya children reflects the political and economic opportunities encountered by Maya refugees living in the United States. At the same time, Maya children remained shorter than the children of the other U.S. ethnic groups living in the same town. Bogin and Loucky concluded that all people live within physical, social, economic, and political environments that have powerful effects on human biology. Although little can be done to alter the physical environment, the political and economic environment can be changed.

Across these biocultural perspectives, the emphasis ranges from hominid evolution to reproductive success within contemporary populations, to biocultural interactions and genetic, developmental or physiological adaptations, to social power relationships. The biocultural perspective applied in this book shares commonalities with all of these approaches, particularly the ecological model, but I do not adopt one point of view exclusively. The topic of menopause is so broad that like the paleoanthropologists, I want to know when menopause first appeared in our evolutionary record. Like the adaptationists, I wonder if reproductive success had a role in the evolution of menopause through natural selection. And like those who employ an ecological model, I find that framework useful for thinking about the influence of diet and health-related behaviors on symptom experience.

The Treatment of Culture in Biocultural Research

Across all of these frameworks, the effects or "artifacts" of culture are most often treated as something that can be measured (the complexity of tools, the presence or absence of water taps in a village, the deprivation of war, "lifestyle incongruity," "social power," economic stress and so on). Other measurable artifacts of culture include medical interventions, attitudes about aging, birth control policy, smoking practices, diet preferences, patterns of breastfeeding, and the socially appropriate timing of motherhood. Measurement of such particulars allows the collection of data that are both meaningful for informants and amenable to cross-cultural comparison (Browner, Ortiz de Montellano, and Rubel 1988).[12]

This emphasis on the measurement of artifacts (things) or standards of behavior (norms) is different from the ways in which culture is understood in other subdisciplines of anthropology and, consequently, in many studies of menopause. For example, with occasional exceptions (such as Worthman 1999), biocultural perspectives generally do not address the concept of "embodiment," a notion that emphasizes the inseparability of the biological and social body, so that the physical body reflects its social context (Csordas 1994; Edgewater 1999; Hinton 1999; Rothfield 1997). Nor, within the biocultural perspective, is there a general comfort with "discourses" about or "dialectics" between biology and culture (Lock 1993).

Researchers who use the biocultural perspective as their theoretical framework are typically comfortable with the idea that there are facts about the world to be uncovered. They much less frequently explore the construction of facts "as a result of interaction between researcher with the subject of research" (Lock and Scheper-Hughes 1996:42). Even when these ideas—facts as real, facts as constructed—are brought together within one interesting volume (Pollard and Hyatt 1999), the chapters remain quite separate.

Although culture, in a biocultural perspective, is often treated as something that can be measured, there is a recognition that cultural ideologies, norms, and meanings shape the measurable variable. In general, however, biocultural anthropologists are measuring the outcome, not the meaning. For example, in Mali breasts are perceived "as existing for the sole purpose of feeding children," and consequently women are able to breastfeed freely (Dettwyler 1995b:171). In the United States, breasts are defined primarily as sex objects, and therefore breasts are not freely exposed and breastfeeding is more often done in private. Cultural norms thus affect the frequency with which infants can be breastfed, and breastfeeding frequency has physiological consequences for both the mother and the child (Stuart-Macadam 1995).

Culture in biocultural research is also generally treated as separate from and external to the physical body. Culture is public, created, contested, and shared through learning. Behaviors associated with culture, such as forms of marriage (Durham 1991), can be measured and modeled as analogous to the forces of biological evolution, in the sense that change occurs through invention (analogous to mutation), diffusion (analogous to gene flow), random loss of information (analogous to genetic drift), and the cultural selection of particular ideas (not always "good" ideas or adaptive ideas, but particular ideas). Predictive models can be constructed, variables measured, and hypotheses tested.

In biocultural models, cultural variables (that is, artifacts and behaviors) and biological variables are both considered. For example, which is more important in explaining hot flashes among women at midlife in Puebla, Mexico: marital status (single, married, living together, divorced, widowed) or estrogen levels? In Puebla, marital status—a measurable variable—is an effect of culture. It is greatly influenced by the ideologies of the Catholic church (divorced people, for example, cannot participate in communion). Marital status is also influenced by the cultural ideal of the nuclear family, and the cultural acceptance of second families among men who will not (for religious or family reasons) divorce their first wives. By contrast, estrogen levels are influenced by the number of follicles developing within the ovary during any particular month.

In Puebla, women who had never married reported significantly fewer hot flashes during the two weeks prior to interview (39 percent) compared with married women (52 percent). The lowest rate of hot flashes (29 percent) was among single women with no children. The highest rate of hot flashes (67 percent) was among married women with no children.[13] Marriage can be very stressful for women in Puebla, and since divorce is frequently not a real option, there is often no way out of a difficult relationship. The resultant unhappiness may be one reason why married women report more uncomfortable physical symptoms at menopause than do single women. Does marital stress translate into neurochemical changes that in turn influence the hypothalamic-pituitary-ovarian axis and result in a higher frequency of hot flashes? This working hypothesis is made possible by the biocultural approach.

With regard to estrogen levels, it appears that postmenopausal women (who are assumed to have lower levels of estrogen than premenopausal women) are more likely to have hot flashes. During the two weeks prior to interview, naturally postmenopausal women were more likely to report hot flashes compared with premenopausal women (57 percent versus 38 percent). In logistic regression analyses (where marital status and menstrual status were examined together in relation to hot flash experience), menopause status was a stronger predictor of hot flash experience compared with marital status. Does that mean that biology will always trump culture? No. The biocultural approach concerns the intertwining of biology and culture, not the triumph of one over the other. It means considering both marriage and menopause status when seeking to explain hot flash frequency.

The Biocultural Approach to Menopause

The biocultural perspective provides a tool kit of analyses for the many different questions raised with regard to the evolution of menopause, variation in age at menopause, and variation in symptoms associated with menopause. The approach is a particularly appropriate framework for the study of menopause for a number of reasons. First, a biocultural perspective recognizes that humans are a product of a long evolutionary history. Across animal species, menopause and postreproductive life are not common characteristics. Most animals die before they cease their ability to reproduce; only human females, not males, have evolved a species-wide cessation of reproductive capacity and prolonged period of post-reproductive life. An understanding of how menopause has evolved sets the stage for examining widely shared aspects of biology and behavior across all humans.

Second, a biocultural perspective allows us to examine the genetic, developmental, and environmental processes that bring about human variation. Information relevant to the study of menopause spans biological levels, from particular genes to entire species. The study of menopause includes analyses of genetic polymorphisms in relation to age at menopause (Cramer et al. 1989); autopsy (Block 1952) and ultrasound studies of ovarian follicular stores (Flaws et al. 2000, 2001); longitudinal and cross-sectional studies of hormonal change (Rannevik et al. 1995); laboratory studies of hot flash physiology (Freedman 2000a); studies of hot flash frequencies across a nation (Avis et al. 1993, 2001) and the world (Boulet et al. 1994; Sievert and Flanagan 2005); and cross-species studies of the length of postreproductive life (Pavelka and Fedigan 1991, 1999).

Third, a biocultural perspective can be used to demonstrate how continuous, normally distributed physiological variation is subject to culturally specific clinical segmentation. Biomedicine defines the boundaries of normal; however, the cutoffs between normal and pathological vary by culture. With regard to menopause, the cutoff between premature ovarian failure and a clinically normal menopause at age forty is arbitrary, since it may not be applicable across all cultures.

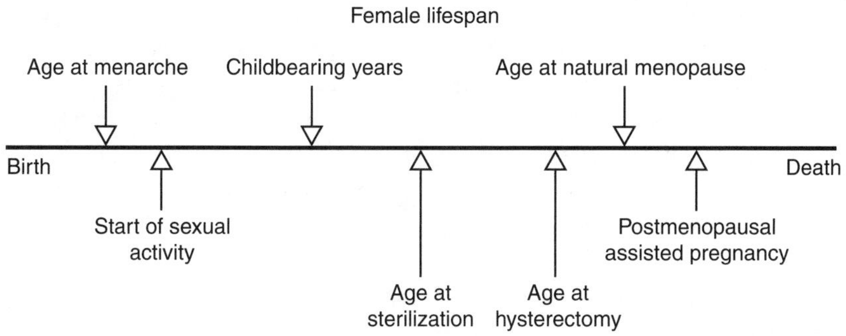

Female lifespan

Age at menarche   Childbearing years   Age at natural menopause

Birth   Death

Start of sexual   Postmenopausal
activity   assisted pregnancy

Age at   Age at
sterilization   hysterectomy

FIGURE 1.7 Cultural and biological boundaries on female reproduction. The vertical arrows slide up and down the female lifespan in culture-specific ways. For example, sometimes sexual activity begins before menarche. Age at menopause can slide down to forty-two or up to fifty-eight, and so on.

Fourth, the biocultural perspective fosters the recognition that there are cultural as well as biological boundaries on female reproduction (figure 1.7). Social attitudes as well as technological innovation can permanently curtail or temporarily prolong the ability to conceive and/or give birth. Terminal abstinence—that is, the practice of stopping sexual relations when one becomes a grandmother (Cavalli-Sforza 1983)—effectively brings about an end to fertility, but not menstruation. Tubal ligation also brings about an end to fertility, but not menstruation. In contrast, a hysterectomy can end menstruation, but leave functioning ovaries intact. A biocultural perspective allows us to consider the ways in which social values and biomedicine complicate the relationship between the end of fertility and cessation of menses.

The Lifespan Approach

The biocultural perspective acknowledges the enmeshed complexity of biology, behavior, attitudes, medicine, and the physical environment. The relationships are seldom direct and there are often confounding factors to consider. The ways in which culture (behavior, attitudes, medicine, physical environment) can influence the fundamental biological basis of menopause are best seen from a lifespan approach (Kuh and Hardy 2002; Leidy 1996a).

The lifespan approach follows biological, sociocultural, and psychological trajectories across time (Elder 1985; Riley 1979; Sorensen, Weinart, and Sherrod 1986) with the conviction that "only the entire lifespan can serve as a satisfactory frame of reference" (Filipp and Olbrich 1986:347–348). Within the lifespan, events and transitions are temporally arranged so that the study of development or aging is "essentially a study of the sequence of events . . . in which earlier events condition later events" (Harris 1987:21–22). Along life's trajectories, menopause can function as a cumulative or a predictive event. It is cumulative in the sense that menopause follows, for example, thirty-two years of smoking and damage to the developing oocytes (resulting in an earlier age at menopause). It is predictive in the sense that age at menopause can be used in population-level models to predict risk of breast cancer or even age at death. In a study of Seventh-Day Adventists, the odds of death decreased as age at natural menopause increased, up to the age of fifty-five (Snowdon 1990; Snowden et al. 1989). Age at natural menopause appeared to predict age at death, at least during the course of the study period. A similar finding was recently reported by researchers in the Netherlands (Ossewaarde et al. 2005).

Age at menopause is set by the number of oocytes (eggs) created by mitosis during prenatal development, and by the rate of oocyte loss through follicular atresia (degeneration) across the lifespan—from the fifth month in utero until the fifth or sixth decade of life. A lifespan perspective is, therefore, consistent with the biology of menopause. For instance, if a mother smokes, one could hypothesize that the store of eggs formed in her daughter's fetal ovaries may be compromised and her daughter may experience menopause at age forty-seven rather than forty-nine. A lifespan approach has been applied to demonstrate a negative correlation in age at menarche and age at menopause in a nutritionally stressed Blackfeet population (Johnston 2001), and a positive correlation in age at menarche and age at menopause among first-generation Hispanic immigrants to the United States (Leidy 1998). A lifespan perspective encourages the formation and testing of hypotheses and questions that stretch across time. For example, does a woman who sleeps with a man for twenty years have more regular periods and, relatedly, a later age at menopause? (The answer appears to be yes; Sievert, Waddle, and Canali 2001.)

Difficulties in applying the lifespan perspective arise both from its overwhelming holism (Silverman 1987) and from the long stretch of time between an attribute of interest (such as oocyte development in utero or childhood nutrition) and menopause, fifty years later. Application of a lifespan approach requires either a prospective, longitudinal study design (and long-lived researchers) or, less valid, a reliance on recalled data in retrospective studies. However, by looking at widely spaced behaviors or biological events, new patterns of constancy and change (Brim and Kagan 1980; Elder 1985), correlations (Leidy 1996b), and risks (Scholl, Hediger, and Schall 1996) can be identified.

For example, in my study of menopause carried out in upstate New York in 1989–1990, I asked women if they had ever experienced a variety of symptoms in association with menstruation (table 1.4) in order to identify possible correlations between recalled menstrual symptoms and the experience of menopausal symptoms later in life. As might be expected, I found strong, positive correlations between headaches with menstruation and headaches at menopause; and between mood swings with menstruation and irritability or mood changes at

TABLE 1.4

Symptom Experience with Menstruation (in Percent)

Symptom Experience	Upstate New York	Puebla, Mexico	Asunción, Paraguay
Bloating	94		
Cramps	93	54	48
Breast tenderness	89		
Mood swings	88	12	28
Headaches	69		
Leg cramps	47		

Source: New York data: Leidy (1996c). Mexico and Paraguay data unpublished.

Note: In Puebla and Asunción, researchers asked directly only about menstrual cramps and mood changes. Women were asked to volunteer any other symptoms that occurred before or during menstruation.

menopause. Of greater interest, I found that menstrual cramps and menopausal hot flashes were significantly related.

In a linear model only abdominal cramps and leg cramps during the menstrual cycle predicted hot flashes at menopause. In other words, having experienced cramps with menstruation during younger years was a significant predictor of hot flashes with menopause during midlife, but irritability or mood swings with menstruation did not predict hot flashes. In contrast, menstrual bloating, breast tenderness, and mood swings (but not cramps) with menstruation were significant predictors of later, menopausal irritability and mood changes (Leidy 1996c).

The association between a history of menstrual cramps and menopausal hot flashes has also been shown in Australia (Dennerstein et al. 1993), Britain (M. Hunter 1992), and Sweden (Holte and Mikkelsen 1991). Similarly, in Puebla, Mexico, menstrual cramps were significantly associated with hot flashes at midlife, so that among women with a history of cramps, 57 percent reported hot flashes; among women with no history of cramps, 48 percent reported hot flashes ($p < .01$) (Leidy Sievert 2003).

In Asunción, Paraguay, women who recalled the experience of cramps with menstruation ($n = 220$) were also more likely to report hot flashes with menopause, compared with women who did not experience cramps with menstruation ($n = 240$) (55 percent versus 38 percent, $p < .01$). There was no similar relationship between having cramps and feelings of sadness at midlife. These similar findings across a variety of cultures suggest that whatever the explanation for the pattern of correlation between symptom experience with menstruation and at menopause (physiology or personality), it is not unique to upstate New York.

The lifespan perspective allows for investigations across widely spaced events; however, like the biocultural approach, the lifespan perspective is a paradigm or general orientation, not a theory (Baltes and Schaie 1973; Brim and Kagan 1980). According to Bernice Neugarten, the lifespan perspective was first adopted by cultural anthropologists interested in age grading and life histories. Then personality psychologists and developmental psychologists embarked on "studies of lives." Finally, sociologists began their work, at times in collaboration with historians (Neugarten 1988). That the lifespan serves as an organizational framework across a number of disciplines is evidenced by differences in vocabulary. For example, the *life history* approach glosses over intraspecies variation in lifespan traits to better demonstrate variation across species (Caro et al. 1995; Gage 1998; Partridge and Harvey 1988; Pavelka and Fedigan 1991). The *life cycle* approach is similar to the life history approach in that the lifespan is described as a series of distinct, bounded stages (Goodfriend and Christie 1988); however, the life cycle perspective allows for variation in lifespan events and transitions.

In the *life course* perspective of sociology, development and aging are understood to form a continuous process from birth to death (Riley 1986) and, in contrast to the life cycle approach, rigid age categories and developmental stages are rejected in favor of identifying patterns, sequences, and correlations across the lifespan (Brettell 2002; Harris 1987; Neugarten 1969). Biological transitions or events, such as birth, weaning, menarche, or menopause cannot be dismissed, as they are essential for cross-category comparisons.

Across the lifespan, time may be perceived to be absolute or relational (Benjamin 1966). For example, to compare age at menopause among populations, menopause must be placed on a linear, chronological, absolute scale. In contrast, relational time can seem to "speed up" or "slow down"; the awareness of time is relative to changing events. In relational time, the significance of a woman's age at menopause may vary in association with different clocks—biological, social, professional, or spiritual (Cartwright 1987). Each trajectory of the lifespan has its own time table so that women can perceive the timing of menopause to be "on time" or "off time" (Neugarten and Datan 1973) in relation to biological or sociocultural events.

In upstate New York, for example, I asked women who were naturally postmenopausal whether or not they "were ready for the end of menstruation." Ninety-three percent said "yes," and 98 percent said that they were ready to stop having children. In contrast to this apparent acceptance of the inevitable, table 1.5 illustrates how the timing of menopause was characterized by naturally postmenopausal women and also by women who underwent menopause by

TABLE 1.5

Characterization of the Timing of Menopause in Upstate New York

Timing of Menopause	Naturally Postmenopausal Women		Postmenopausal by Hysterectomy	
	Frequency (n = 114)	Mean Age at Menopause (S.D.) (n = 98)	Frequency (n = 29)	Mean Age at Hysterectomy (S.D.) (n = 29)
"Early"	18%	44.5 (5.6)	66%	39.7 (7.5)
"On time"	63	50.2 (2.9)	21	44.0 (4.8)
"Late"	13	52.3 (4.9)	0	
"Don't know"	5	49.5 (2.3)	14	35.8 (10.9)

Source: Leidy (1991).

hysterectomy. More women who experienced menopause by hysterectomy said that their menopause was "early"; none said that their menopause was "late." However, it is too easy to say that women with earlier chronological ages at menopause were more likely to characterize their menopause as "early." As standard deviations illustrate, there is variation around the mean. Naturally postmenopausal women who said their menopause was "early" were as old as fifty-one at the time of their last menstrual period. Among women who considered menopause to be "on time," eleven women reported menopause from ages fifty-three to fifty-eight. In contrast, one woman who described menopause as "late" said her last menstrual period was at age thirty-seven (Leidy 1991).

Further investigation showed that each woman created her own time scale of average or expected ages at menopause, and each scale was constructed, in part, through comparisons with other women. For example, in upstate New York, women who experienced menopause before what they believed to be the average age for menopause (anywhere from thirty-five to fifty-eight years of age) described the timing of their menopause as "early" more often than "on time" or "late." It didn't matter whether or not they were right in a demographic sense. What they believed to be the age norm (Neugarten 1969) for menopause influenced how they described the timing of their own last menstrual period. Among women who experienced what they believed to be an average age at menopause, 88 percent said their menopause was "on time"—even though their ages at menopause ranged from forty-five to fifty-five (Leidy 1991).

In addition to chronological scales, some women used family stage as a consideration in deciding whether their menopause was "early," "on time," or "late." One participant noted that she was ready for the end of menstruation because "I was divorced." A forty-one-year-old participant commented that menopause should occur at forty-five because "I think that women are then becoming too old/tired to care for new babies and children." A fifty-eight-year-old respondent said that she wished menopause had occurred at fifty because "it is time to become a grandmother rather than a new mother." Other women referred to their occupational role. For example, one forty-three-year-old premenopausal woman suggested that periods should stop between forty-eight and fifty because that is "close to retirement." A fifty-three-year-old postmenopausal woman noted that because of career demands she would have liked menopause to occur at fifty (instead of fifty-one) because it was "one less thing to cope with!" (Leidy 1991).

Finally, women used a third scale, that of gynecologic age. In response to the question, "When would you like your periods to stop?" a forty-two-year-old women said, "Thirty-two years is enough!" Explained one forty-six-year-old woman, "Forty years is enough! I think it would be really neat to have menopause at a set number of years after beginning your period. Then you would know when menopause would happen" (Leidy 1991). The extent to which women consciously add up their years of menstruation is unknown; however, there was a statistically significant difference among postmenopausal women with a reproductive span of less than thirty-four years who were more likely to describe their menopause as "early" (43 percent) or "on time" (53 percent) compared with women with a reproductive span of thirty-four to forty years who were more likely to say that their menopause was "on time" (77 percent), compared with women with a reproductive span of more than forty years who were more likely to say that their menopause was "on time" (50 percent) or "late" (50 percent) ($p < .01$).[14]

In the lifespan approach the biological, social, and psychological trajectories are viewed as lifelong (Baltes and Schaie 1973; Mercer, Nichols, and Doyle 1989; Riley, Abeles, and Teitelbaum 1982) and "no single stage of a person's life . . . can be understood apart from its antecedents and consequences" (Riley 1979:4). For example, a woman will not view menopause as a marker of the end of fertility if she has undergone a tubal ligation or other type of sterilization. In Puebla, we found that 42.5 percent of women had undergone a tubal ligation at an average age of thirty-three years (Sievert 2003).[15] Figure 1.8 shows the number of women who underwent sterilization at each age (triangles), the number of women who underwent hysterectomy at each age (open circles), and the number of women who underwent a natural menopause at each age (solid circles). From a lifespan perspective, tubal ligations bring about an end to fertility prior to natural menopause. Hysterectomies bring about an end to fertility (unless there has already been a sterilization procedure) and bring about an end to menstruation prior to natural menopause. Natural menopause marks the

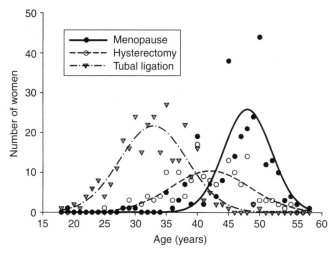

FIGURE 1.8 Ages at tubal ligation, hysterectomy, and natural menopause in Puebla, Mexico. Courtesy of Paul R. Sievert.

end of fertility (unless there has already been a sterilization procedure or hysterectomy) and is the end of menstruation (unless there has already been a hysterectomy).

Midlife is a point of cumulation, just like young adulthood, childhood, and even infancy. Each woman accumulates a biological as well as a social history. In turn, biological insults, repairs, and behaviors at midlife will have even later biological and social consequences. This lifespan approach is, a fitting complement to the biocultural perspective.

CHAPTER TWO

The Biological Basis of Menopause

Background Endocrinology

One factor that inhibits a biocultural approach to any topic is the scientific literacy required to make sense of the relevant underlying biology. For readers not familiar with the language of reproductive biology, this section expands on the biological details with more terms and definitions.

The hypothalamus, the pituitary, and the ovaries maintain menstrual cycles in premenopausal women. These organs are part of the endocrine or hormonal system. The organs of the endocrine system communicate with one another, and with other organs and tissues. Hormones are messengers that carry chemical information to receptors which are designed to interpret and act on specific messages. For example, the hormone estrogen is produced within the ovary and sent, via the bloodstream, to estrogen receptors in breast, bone, adipose (fat), vaginal, cervical, uterine, and skin tissues (Merry and Holehan 1994; Whitehead, Whitcroft, and Hilliard 1993).[1]

Within the brain, the hypothalamus and pituitary gland communicate closely and exert control over the function of endocrine glands, including the ovaries, as well as over a range of physiologic activities such as the regulation of food intake and body temperature. Changes in the ability to control body temperature are implicated in the etiology (causation) of hot flashes, which are discussed in more detail in Chapter Six.

In the brain, the hypothalamus transmits a hormone called Gonadotropin Releasing Hormone (GnRH) directly to the anterior pituitary. This transmission occurs in pulses. Neurotransmitters such as catecholamines (for example, norepinephrine and dopamine), serotonin, and endorphin modify the secretion of GnRH (Dobson et al. 2003; Ferin, Van Vugt, and Wardlaw 1984; Genazzani et al. 2000; Herbison 1997; Kaiser, Morley, and Korenman 1993; Meites et al. 1982). Norepinephrine is a neurotransmitter that stimulates a fight-or-flight reaction

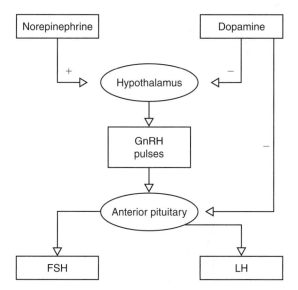

FIGURE 2.1 Neurotransmitters and GnRH release.

Redrawn from Speroff, Glass, and Kase (1999:170).

(such as increases in heart rate and blood pressure) in response to short-term stress. As figure 2.1 shows, brain norepinephrine facilitates GnRH release. We are interested in brain norepinephrine levels because they rise before and during hot flashes (Freedman and Woodward 1992).

Dopamine is a precursor of norepinephrine, but also functions as a neurotransmitter by itself. Dopamine is involved in the control of movement (a lack of dopamine is associated with Parkinson's disease) and in feelings of enjoyment. Dopamine suppresses GnRH release (Speroff, Glass, and Kase 1999). The effect of serotonin is less well understood. Serotonin is now widely recognized for the role it plays in the biochemistry of depression and anxiety. Most people have heard of antidepressants, such as Prozac, which are selective serotonin reuptake inhibitors, or SSRIs. The activity of neurotransmitters is altered by age (Wise et al. 1997), as well as by environmental stimuli (Meites and Lu 1994), including stress. The neuroendocrine system is thus a complex system of communication, affecting multiple areas of physiological function at once.

The anterior pituitary, because of its important role in communicating and directing physiological changes throughout the body, is richly vascularized (Greenspan and Baxter 1994:66), meaning that it is laced with blood vessels to better monitor and send hormonal signals. Receptors in the anterior pituitary sense the pulse frequency and amplitude of GnRH and direct the production of two gonadotropins, follicle stimulating hormone (FSH; see table 1.1). and luteinizing hormone (LH).[2] Both hormones are critical to the reproductive process. FSH stimulates follicle development and stimulates ovulation. LH also stimulates ovulation and then the development of the corpus luteum, the progesterone-secreting endocrine gland that forms from the ruptured follicle.

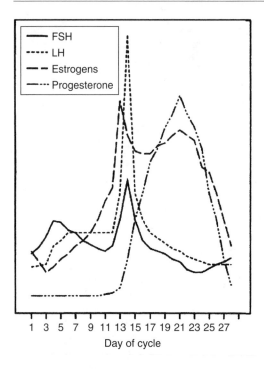

FIGURE 2.2 Levels of LH, FSH, total estrogens, and progesterone across the menstrual cycle. Hormones are presented as percent maximum secretion. Redrawn from Schnatz (1985:7).

Although FSH and LH are both stimulated by GnRH, the two hormones are under separate regulatory control. For example, women have higher levels of FSH relative to levels of LH during the follicular phase of menstrual cycles (figure 2.2). Also, as will be discussed below, there is an earlier rise in FSH levels prior to menopause; there is also an age-related loss of concordance between LH and FSH pulses (Backstrom et al. 1982; Burger et al. 1998; Channing et al. 1985; Genazzani et al. 1997; Lee et al. 1988; Rannevik et al. 1995).

Within the ovaries, FSH and LH stimulate oogenesis (the development of the egg), follicular growth (follicles surround and nourish the egg), and ovarian production of estrogens, progesterone, inhibins (hormones that inhibit FSH production) and small amounts of androgens (hormones such as testosterone that are more frequently associated with males). A review of follicle development will help to make better sense of these functions of FSH and LH.

In a five- to six-week-old human female embryo, primordial germ cells originate in the wall of the yolk sac and migrate into the embryo where the fetus's ovaries will eventually develop (Moore 1988). Sex cells (eggs) thus have a different embryological origin (the yolk sac) than do the other tissues of the body. These germ cells develop into oogonia which, from the eleventh to twelfth week onward, form oocytes through mitosis (cellular duplication) (T. G. Baker 1986; Crisp 1992; Moore 1988). As noted earlier, oocyte formation ceases by the time a human fetus is five months old (T. G. Baker 1986). Unlike men, who continue to make sex cells (sperm) well into their later years, women do not make sex cells (oocytes) past their fifth month in utero (unless we discover surprising new evidence that, like some mice, humans are capable of producing eggs after birth (Johnson et al. 2004)). The number of oocytes formed prior to birth determines, in part, a woman's age at menopause, as will be discussed more fully in Chapter Four.

At about sixteen weeks in utero, oocytes are surrounded by a layer of flattened granulosa cells (Moore 1988). At this stage of development, these units are now called primordial follicles. Oocytes that remain naked, without a layer of granulosa cells, degenerate (Weir and Rowlands 1977). This fact may explain the rapid decline in oocyte numbers from the peak of seven million to the approximately two million oocytes present at birth. During menstrual cycles, later in life, primordial follicles act as a pool from which all developing follicles emerge (Peters and McNatty 1980).

Across the lifespan, from twenty-six weeks in utero until menopause, primordial follicles develop into preantral, then antral, follicles with granulosa and theca cellular envelopes (figure 1.2) (C. R. Martin 1985; Peters and McNatty 1980; Reynaud et al. 2004). Granulosa and theca cells function to nourish the oocyte. They also produce hormones, including estrogen. The number of antral follicles in the ovary are correlated with chronological age and probably reflect the size of the reserve pool of primordial follicles (Scheffer et al. 1999). As follicles go through their developmental sequence, they produce increasing amounts of estrogen and inhibin. Inhibin reduces the secretion of FSH in the pituitary gland. Following ovulation, the follicle becomes a corpus luteum, secreting large amounts of progesterone. Follicular development is responsible for the pattern of changes in hormone levels across the menstrual cycle, as seen earlier in figure 2.2.

Follicles at all stages of development are present in the ovaries during the reproductive years. Although follicular development can lead to ovulation, ovulation accounts for very few of the follicles lost across a woman's lifespan. Instead, 99.9 percent of all oocytes disappear from the ovary through the degenerative process of atresia, not ovulation (Finch and Gosden 1986; Peters and McNatty 1980). Researchers interested in what happens at the end of a woman's reproductive years must understand these developmentally early processes, as the rate of follicle loss across the lifespan also determines, in part, a woman's age at menopause.

Various hormones rise, fall, and interact during the menstrual cycle. FSH from the pituitary binds to specific hormone receptors on the membrane of the granulosa cells of the ovarian follicle. LH binds to receptors on the membranes of both granulosa and theca cells of the ovarian follicle (figure 2.3). Together, FSH and LH stimulate the granulosa cells of the ovarian follicle to form estradiol (a potent estrogen) through the conversion of an androgen (androstenedione) derived from the theca cells (Erickson 2000). Androstenedione also bears

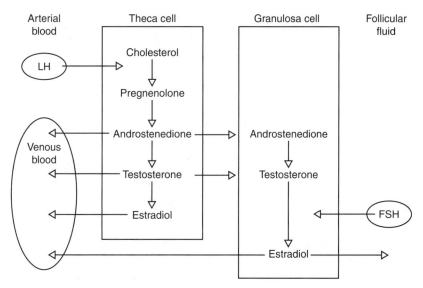

FIGURE 2.3 A model of the process by which FSH and LH stimulate the production of estradiol within ovarian follicles. LH (left) and FSH (right) stimulate the production of estradiol from cholesterol by way of androstenedione and testosterone (in theca cells) and from androstenedione by way of testosterone (in granulosa cells).

Modified from Peters and McNatty (1980).

mention (if not memorization) because this hormone is also converted to estrone (a weak estrogen) by fat and muscle tissue throughout the body.

FSH levels (see figure 2.2) rise at the end of the luteal phase (or second half) of one menstrual cycle and through the first week of the follicular phase of the next cycle. During this rise in FSH, a dominant follicle is selected for ovulation from the pool of antral follicles. As the dominant follicle develops, estrogen and inhibin A are produced and their levels in the bloodstream rise. Maximum rates of estrogen production are attained just before ovulation. The high level of estrogen triggers preovulatory surges of FSH and LH. (This is the one time that estrogen has a positive feedback effect on the pituitary hormones.) The surge of FSH and LH will ultimately trigger the release of the egg from the preovulatory follicle. The egg will enter the fallopian tube and make its way to the uterus. Along the way, it may be fertilized by a sperm.

There are two types of inhibin secreted by the ovary. Inhibin A, as we have seen, is primarily a product of the dominant follicle. Levels of inhibin A rise with the preovulatory rise in estradiol, then peak during the luteal phase (as it continues to be produced by the corpus luteum). Inhibin B is the product of the pool of growing follicles. There is an early rise of inhibin B during the follicular phase, a midcycle peak, then levels fall (Burger et al. 2002).

Throughout the reproductive phase of life, hormones produced in the ovaries—estrogen, progesterone, and inhibin—send feedback signals to the brain, regulating the secretion of FSH and LH (Channing et al. 1985; Guraya 1985; Merry and Holehan 1994; Wood 1994). Although both inhibins and estradiol exert negative feedback effects on pituitary FSH and LH secretion, it is the fall in inhibin B levels that is generally understood to be the cause of the rise in FSH levels during the late perimenopause transition (Burger et al. 2002). When there isn't enough inhibin B produced because the number of follicles in the ovary is too small, then FSH is freed from inhibin's control and starts to rise (table 1.1). The threshold number of ovarian follicles needed to maintain monthly hormonal cycles also determines, in part, a woman's age at menopause.

Across the female lifespan, there is thus a rapid increase and then a slow loss in the number of follicles. The hypothalamus, pituitary, and ovaries communicate via hormonal messengers to establish the menstrual cycle. We have also noted the developmental sequence of primordial to preantral to antral to preovulatory follicles. Menopause occurs when the number of ovarian follicles drops below the threshold number needed to maintain monthly hormonal cycles.

The Menopause Transition

There is also endocrinology specific to the menopause transition. Sometimes people are surprised to learn that women continue to experience cyclic hormonal fluctuations well beyond the cessation of menstruation. These changes in hormone levels, due to continued follicular development within the ovary, can still be associated with changes in mood, breast tenderness, or fluid retention (bloating), even though a woman is no longer menstruating. Although menstrual cycles and the ability to become pregnant may have come to an end, primordial follicles continue to exist in the ovaries of women over the age of fifty (Costoff and Mahesh 1975; Novak 1970). Darryl Holman, Kathleen O'Connor, and colleagues showed that these primordial follicles occasionally begin to grow even though menstruation has stopped. In their study, 108 participants of the Tremin Research Program, aged twenty-seven to sixty, contributed urine specimens and menstrual diaries for six months. Fifty participants reported no menstrual bleeding and demonstrated elevated FSH concentrations. Of these, thirteen exhibited "unambiguous evidence" of follicular development, as assessed by at least a threefold gradual rise followed by a decline in a metabolite of estradiol (estrone-3-glucuronide). There was follicular development, but no evidence of ovulation or menses (Holman, Wood, and Campbell 2002).

Although follicular development may thus continue for a time after the cessation of menses, it is still correct to say that the trigger for menopause appears to be in the ovaries (Bennett and Whitehead 1983).[3] As menopause approaches, the sequence of hormonal feedback (figure 2.2) remains the same, but hormonal levels are modified with age. Some researchers have found that premenopausal women complain of hot flashes or night sweats right before the start of menstruation, even though their menstrual cycles are regular and menopause may seem to be a long way off (Guthrie et al. 1996; Hahn, Wong, and Reid 1998). These premenopausal hot flashes may occur as a result of an age-related decline in estrogen levels during the luteal (postovulation) phase.

Also as menopause approaches, the length of the follicular phase (prior to ovulation) is shortened and FSH levels increase, particularly during the early follicular phase (Lee et al. 1988; Sherman 1987). This is the basis for the Menocheck at-home test discussed in Chapter One. Because of the increase in FSH, one staging system for classifying women as either reproductive, in the menopause transition, or postmenopausal is based on menstrual cycle regularity and increased levels of this hormone (Soules et al. 2001; Utian 2001). This staging system, developed in July 2001 by the Stages of Reproductive Aging Workshop (STRAW), will be discussed in greater detail in Chapter Four. The age-related increase in FSH that occurs before the age-related increase of LH is thought to be the result of lower inhibin B secretion by the ovaries (Burger et al. 1998, 2002).

Significant increases in serum FSH and LH begin about five years prior to menopause (Rannevik et al. 1995), although hormonal changes come and go and vary greatly with age (Metcalf, Donald, and Livesey 1981; Reame et al. 1996). There is no definitive hormonal marker for the inception of "perimenopause" (Santoro 1996). However, as the ovarian follicular supply is exhausted, there is a marked decrease in estradiol and estrone and FSH and LH remain elevated (Longcope et al. 1986). Figure 2.4 summarizes the hormonal changes of 160 women who were observed for seven to twelve years through their menopausal transition. The FSH levels listed in table 1.1 are shown on this graph, along with LH, estradiol, and estrone levels. Mean age at menopause for this Swedish population was 52.1 years, ranging from 48.3 to 57.4 years (Rannevik et al. 1995:107).

After menopause, serum levels of LH and FSH decline but remain higher than premenopausal levels (Genazzani et al. 1997). There is a continued decline in levels of estradiol and estrone, as shown in figure 2.4. Estradiol, the most physiologically active estrogen, declines most markedly. Estrone continues to be produced through the conversion of androstenedione to estrone in muscle, adipose, and other tissues. This production of estrone by fat tissue is one reason why researchers have expected to find fewer hot flashes in heavier women (Campagnoli et al. 1981; Erlik, Meldrum, and Judd 1982; Huerta et al. 1995; Schwingl, Hulka, and Harlow 1994); however, the results have not always been consistent on this point (Carpenter et al. 1998; Chiechi et al. 1997; den Tonkelaar, Seidell, and van Noord 1996; Freeman et al. 2001; Gold et al. 2000; Sternfeld, Quesenberry, and Husson 1999; Wilbur et al. 1998).

In summary, female reproductive senescence in humans is due to the loss of ovarian follicles across time. Age at menopause is thus determined by the

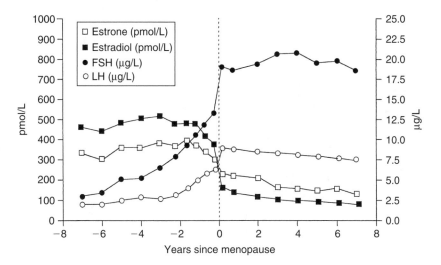

FIGURE 2.4 Changes in FSH, LH, estradiol, and estrone levels among women followed longitudinally through the menopausal transition.

Reprinted from *Maturitas,* 21, Rannevik et al., A longitudinal study of the perimenopausal transition: altered profiles of steroid and pituitary hormones, SHBG, and bone mineral density, 103–113, © 1995, and with permission from Elsevier, and from *Reproductive Ecology and Human Evolution,* edited by Peter T. Ellison, copyright © 2001 by Transaction Publishers. Reprinted by permission of the publisher.

number of oocytes formed in the female ovary by the fifth month of fetal development; by the rate of oocyte loss across the lifespan through the processes of ovulation and degenerative atresia; and by the threshold number of ovarian follicles needed to maintain menstrual cycle regularity (Gosden 1985; Gougeon 1996; Leidy 1994a; Richardson, Senika, and Nelson 1987; Wood 1994). The loss of ovarian follicles results in a decline in inhibin levels and a rise in pituitary hormones, FSH first and foremost. The decline in ovarian estradiol is associated with some negative effects in various target tissues, for example, vaginal dryness (discussed more fully in Chapter Five). At present there is no way to assess "ovarian age," although number of antral follicles (Scheffer et al. 1999), and ovarian volume measured by transvaginal ultrasound technology (Flaws et al. 2000) may allow for an indirect estimation of follicular numbers.

Defining Normal

Human variation is the product of past evolutionary forces and current environmental influences. Prior to the mid-1950s, human variation was the focus of study for investigators wishing to classify human populations into various racial categories (Marks 1995). Currently, the study of human variation seeks to describe

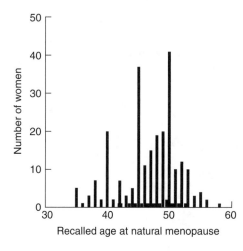

FIGURE 2.5 Recalled ages at natural menopause among women in Puebla, Mexico.

Reprinted from *Human Biology*, 75:2, p. 213, with the permission of Wayne State University Press.

and understand the processes of biologic change (Relethford 2003). Contemporary anthropologists and human biologists are interested in the continuum of human variation across a range of traits. Age at menopause is studied as the outcome of a process of follicle loss—whether the depletion of follicles occurs at age thirty-five or fifty-five. In contrast, biomedical researchers are interested in the assignment of diagnostic categories—normality and pathology.

Figure 2.5 illustrates the range of recalled ages at natural menopause among women in Puebla, Mexico (Sievert and Hautaniemi 2003). Fifty was the most commonly reported age at menopause (also true in western Massachusetts and Asunción, Paraguay), and more women experienced menopause before the age of fifty than after (also true in western Massachusetts and Asunción). Are all of the ages at menopause shown in figure 2.5 "normal"?

Within biomedicine, disease is defined as a deviation from normal functioning, with an emphasis on objective numerical measurement (Hahn 1995). This point of view shapes an understanding of menopause as the end of a normal state—that is, the end of menstruation. The emphasis on numerical measurement leads to the establishment of a cutoff between "premature" menopause (or premature ovarian failure, generally before age forty) and a "normal" age at menopause. The implications of this cutoff will be explored further in Chapter Four; here a few words on the definition of "normal" are appropriate.

In general, biomedical researchers are interested in placing cutoffs along a continuum of variation between normal and pathological. For example, a sample of blood pressures from any population will demonstrate a range of systolic (top number) and diastolic (bottom number) pressures, from very low (for example, 78/54) to very high (for example, 204/112). Many interesting questions arise for human biologists along this continuum. How does blood pressure vary in relation to ethnicity (Brown et al. 1998, 2003), the menstrual cycle (James and

Marion 1994), body mass index (Gerber et al. 1999), or social stress (Dressler 1996)? Medical clinicians, on the other hand, are more interested in differentiating "normal" blood pressure from hypertension (high blood pressure). The criteria to identify hypertension, as formulated by the World Health Organization and the International Society of Hypertension, is either a systolic blood pressure greater than or equal to 140 mm Hg and/or a diastolic blood pressure of greater than or equal to 90 mm Hg (WHO 1999).

Hypertension is a risk factor for a variety of cardiovascular events (heart attack, stroke), so cutoffs help physicians know when to begin treatment. The cutoffs are based on morbidity (sickness) and mortality (death) data; however, the data are interpreted within a culture-specific context of medical standards and treatment protocol. The arbitrary nature of the significance assigned to blood pressure readings was illustrated by Payer's (1988) discussion of German health care in which *hypo*tension (low blood pressure) was treated as a serious health concern. Payer identified eighty-five drugs prescribed for hypotension in Germany at the time of her writing.

Contemporary cross-cultural and historical studies demonstrate further that the cutoffs imposed on human variation to differentiate "normal" from pathological are culture-bound and arbitrary. Several caveats are in order, however. First, human variation is often visible and generally measurable. In other words, while the cutoff is medically established, the existence of human biological variation is not a cultural construct. Second, there are significant health consequences associated with some forms of human variation. Third, the arbitrariness of medical norms is most apparent in the gray areas (such as a diastolic pressure of 90 versus one of 100). If only the extremes are considered (say, diastolic pressure of 160), then it does not seem arbitrary to have some sort of cutoff.

Sometimes it is not the cutoffs that change, but the significance of the pathology. For example, within any population, birth weights, like blood pressure, form a continuum of variation. Babies who are born with low birth weights (less than 5.5 pounds) are at an increased risk for infant mortality. More recently, reinforcing the benefits of a lifespan approach, it has been recognized that low weight at birth is predictive of cardiovascular disease later in life (Barker 1998). Cameron and Demerath (2002) further review diseases that occur later in life and that are associated with low weight at birth.

Sometimes it is recognized that the norms for one country cannot be applied in other populations, so new cutoffs are needed. For example, BMI (kg/m^2) is a measure of fatness that is a risk factor for many diseases, such as diabetes and cardiovascular disease. The World Health Organization recommends a BMI of 25 or over as the cutoff for overweight and a BMI of 30 as the cutoff for obesity (WHO 1995).[4] The arbitrary nature of the cutoffs for BMI has recently been demonstrated by researchers who advocate changing the cutoffs for obesity in China, Singapore, Malaysia, and India to a lower number (Cheng 2003; Deurenberg-Yap

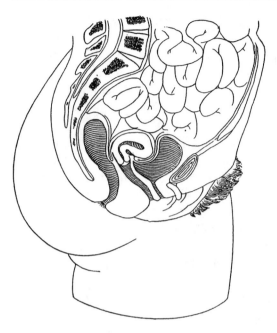

FIGURE 2.6 Nineteenth-century example of uterine displacement. This illustration shows anteflexion of the neck and body of the uterus (Davenport 1898:200). The uterus looks as though it is folded forward in between the bladder on the right and the rectum on the left. The same source has similar illustrations for retroversion and retroflexion of the uterus.

and Deurenberg 2003; Vikram et al. 2003). These populations demonstrate an increased risk of cardiovascular disease at BMI values considered "normal" in other populations. Thus it appears that the "normal" ranges of BMI need to be revised.

A fascinating example of how medical cutoffs change with time is the diagnosis and treatment of uterine displacement. During the nineteenth century and into the early twentieth century, physicians concerned themselves with the degree to which a woman's uterus had tilted forward (anteversion) or backward (retroversion) as in figure 2.6. Physicians developed instruments to measure the extent of displacement and created a host of treatments to keep the uterus in place (Leidy 1994b). Gradually, however, displacement of the uterus was no longer seen as pathological until, except for uterine prolapse, deviation in uterine position became simply a point of conversation during a pelvic exam.

The assumptions of biomedicine shape the cultural context in which menopause occurs. These assumptions (Hahn 1995) include the definition of disease as a deviation from normal functioning (menopause as the end of productive life), an emphasis on objective numerical measurement (menopause before age forty is considered pathological), and a doctrine of specific etiology (menopause understood in terms of estrogen deficiency). The historical focus on the loss of estrogen at the time of menopause influences what are thought to be the typical symptoms associated with menopause (for example, hot flashes rather than bone-muscle-joint pain; Carda et al. 1998).

Missing from this perspective is an appreciation of the evolution of human menopause as, perhaps, an adaptive trait. The relatively new field of Darwinian medicine asks whether or not conditions treated as abnormal or pathological may be reunderstood in adaptive terms (Nesse and Williams 1994; Trevathan, Smith, and McKenna 1999).

The Evolution of Human Menopause

Individual macaques, a common marmoset, a baboon, and one chimpanzee *(Pan paniscus)* have demonstrated endocrinologic (hormonal) and histologic (cellular) changes similar to those of human menopause (Einspanier and Gore 2005; Gould, Flint, and Graham 1981; Hodgen et al. 1977; Lapin et al. 1979; Walker 1995). Chimpanzees in the wild (Nishida, Takasaki, and Takahata 2003) and some free-ranging Japanese macaques (Pavelka and Fedigan 1999; Takahata et al. 1995) have demonstrated postreproductive life. Most reproductive biologists agree, however, that the universal nature of the human menopause is unique among primates, and no other primate experiences such a long period of postreproductive life. As we saw in Chapter One, all human females who live to sixty years of age experience menopause, and they can spend more than half of their maximum lifespan potential in postreproductive life (as was shown in figure 1.1). For example, Jeanne Louise Calment of France lived to the age of 122. If she experienced menopause at fifty years of age, she would have spent more than seventy years in a postreproductive stage of life. Is this adaptive? If evolution through natural selection is driven to maximize reproductive success, how can we explain, in evolutionary terms, such a long postreproductive period?

As touched on above, biological evolution refers to a change in allele frequency within a population (microevolution) or to the development of a new species through the accumulation of many microevolutionary changes (macroevolution). The evolution of contemporary *Homo sapiens* from an earlier hominid species, *Homo erectus*, is an example of macroevolution. The evolution of humans from the last common ancestor that humans shared with the chimpanzee is another example of macroevolution. Evolution tinkers with, reshapes, and builds on ancestral structures and functions. In other words, the physiology and function of our bodies, including menopause, is the product of our phylogeny, our evolutionary history.

To fully understand the evolution of menopause, the timing of menopause, and maybe even the symptoms associated with human menopause, we have to examine the life histories of our closest relatives (other primates), more distant relatives (other mammals), and even more distant relatives (birds, reptiles, amphibians, and fish) (figure 1.5). Here the word "relative" is used to show that, just like family members, we share genetic material with other primates, mammals, even fish. For example, human females need a maximum of four hundred eggs for all the ovulatory cycles of the reproductive years. Rather than just making the four hundred needed, female fetuses produce millions of eggs. This excessive egg production may be viewed as an evolutionary carryover from ancestors that engaged in external fertilization, such as fish (C. R. Martin 1985).

Adaptive Scenarios for the Evolution of Human Menopause

Menopause and/or postreproductive life might be favored by natural selection in a number of ways. First, menopause ensures that mothers are young enough to survive pregnancy, delivery, and the infancy of their offspring. This argument implies that maternal death, more than paternal death, threatens the survival of the youngest offspring, and that "menopause ensures that children are born to mothers likely to live long enough to rear them" (Pollard 1994:214). Because of menopause, women cease childbearing early enough to allow the last child to remain dependent for perhaps fifteen to sixteen years (Lancaster and Lancaster 1983). Hill and Hurtado (1991) used data from the Aché foragers of eastern Paraguay to show that offspring survivorship is low when mothers die in the first five years of the child's life.[5]

Relatedly, pregnancy and childbirth make numerous physiological demands on the mother, and it is thought that, in the context of nutritional stress, the biological resources of older mothers are more severely taxed by the growing fetus than are those of younger mothers. The "*proportion* of available maternal reserves diverted to the fetus will increase with maternal age" (Peacock 1991:375, original emphasis). Moreover, even as the proportion of reserves increases, older mothers are increasingly at risk for negative birth outcomes, including low birth weight and prematurity (Aldous and Edmonson 1993; Fretts et al. 1995). It may simply be adaptive to cease reproducing and invest in offspring already born.

Second, menopause ensures that old, abnormal eggs are not fertilized (Hrdy 1999; C. R. Martin 1985; O'Rourke and Ellison 1993; Pollard 1994). Human oocytes wait in the ovary for fifteen to fifty years prior to ovulation. The increase in risk of fetal loss with maternal age is due, primarily, to an increased incidence of chromosomal aberrations in the eggs of older women (Forbes 1997; Holman et al. 2000; Kline and Levin 1992; Wood 1994). Across mammalian species, the oocytes are stored until ovulation, and this waiting is associated with an age-related increased risk of chromosomal abnormalities (Kohn 1978). Again, rather than risk a compromised pregnancy or birth, it may be adaptive to invest in offspring already born.

Third, the end of menstrual cycles conserves maternal energy. Roberta Hall (2004) combines an explanation for the evolutionary origins of menopause with explanations for the origins of menstruation. The reasoning begins with the observation that high metabolic costs are associated with reproduction, and that therefore opportunities to save energy evolved. Menstrual bleeding saves the energy required to maintain an enriched endometrium (Strassman 1996) and,

Hall proposes, menopause evolved so that energy spent in menstrual cycling could otherwise be used to support offspring survival. In making her argument, Hall draws on an example from Jane Goodall's long-term study of Gombe's chimpanzees. The example concerns Flo, a maternally successful, high-status female.

> The offspring that Flo produced late in her life stressed her to the point that she could not discipline her next-youngest offspring, Flint. The result was that Flo and both offspring died. "If she had not conceived again, all would, I think, have gone well for Flint. But that last pregnancy drained so much strength and energy from Flo's aging body that she was simply not able to wean Flint" (Goodall 1990:193). In effect, Goodall is arguing that menopause would have benefitted Flo and Flint, and if Flint had lived to reproductive age, Flo's inclusive fitness also would have increased. (Hall 2004:93)

Inclusive fitness is a measure of one's contribution to the population gene pool that takes into account not just one's children but one's nieces, nephews, grandchildren, and their children (Hamilton 1966). For example, you share one fourth of your genes with each of your nieces, nephews, and grandchildren; therefore they are part of your evolutionary legacy.

Menopause as an adaptation to aging mothers, aging eggs, and excessive energy expenditure can account for the cessation of fertility; however, none of these arguments explain the extreme length of the human female's postreproductive life. Instead, as noted earlier, many authors have pointed to our long postreproductive life to argue that menopause and postreproductive aging were selected for by the evolutionary benefits gained through grandparenting. This "grandmother hypothesis" is the fourth way in which menopause and/or postreproductive life may have been favored by natural selection. The general argument is that, during human evolution, as offspring dependency increased and more adult care was required, females contributed more genes to the population gene pool by investing in their grandchildren than they could have contributed by continuing to produce children of their own (Alexander 1974; Dawkins 1976; Hamilton 1966; Williams 1957).

The grandmother hypothesis portrays menopause as an advantageous trait within the context of extended families (Donaldson 1984, 1994; Evans 1981; Gaulin 1980; Kirkwood 1985). Despite its broad acceptance, the grandmother hypothesis has been difficult to test with human data (Hames 1984; Hill and Hurtado 1991; Mayer 1982; Peccei 1995; Rogers 1993; Turke 1988). For example, Hill and Hurtado (1991) constructed various demographic models using data from the Aché of Paraguay to estimate the expected benefits and costs of reproductive senescence and concluded that reproductive senescence would not be favored by natural selection, because the grandmother effect is small and most women have few living adult offspring to help. In contrast, Lahdenperä et al. (2004) used Canadian and Finnish samples drawn from eighteenth- and nineteenth-century farming communities, where grandparents resided with or near their offspring, to demonstrate that postreproductive women gained two extra grandchildren for every ten years that they lived beyond age fifty. In Finland, both sons and daughters who had a living, postmenopausal mother had children sooner, at shorter intervals, and more of those children reached adulthood.

Many proponents of the grandmother hypothesis focus not on the early end of fertility but on the evolution of a long, postreproductive life. In these models, emphasis is placed on food foraging by postmenopausal grandmothers. This work is based largely on fieldwork with traditional foragers, the Hadza, who live in the arid savanna woodlands of northern Tanzania (Hawkes, O'Connell, and Blurton Jones 1997). Hawkes and colleagues (1997) argue that if a grandmother feeds a weaned but still dependent grandchild, then the mother can have the next baby sooner. This increases the inclusive fitness of the grandmother. This would imply a selection against somatic senescence (deleterious changes with age in the body); however, ovarian senescence (leading to menopause) would have remained unaffected.[6] As O'Connell, Hawkes, and Blurton Jones (1999) observed, "extended fertility would *not* have been favored as it would have interfered with assistance to grandchildren and the enhanced fecundity at younger ages enjoyed by the daughters of older helpers" (468, original emphasis). O'Connell and colleagues go on to argue that this change in hominid life history traits occurred during the evolution of *Homo erectus.* Their argument is based on archeological, paleontologic, climatic, and contemporary foragers' collection and food processing patterns.

To make things more complicated, some studies have shown that only maternal grandmothers have a positive effect on the survival of grandchildren (Jamison et al. 2002; Voland and Beise 2002), whereas paternal grandmothers and grandfathers are associated with an increased risk of infant death. But maternal grandmothers (mothers of daughters) are also paternal grandmothers (mothers of sons). Peccei (2001) raises some additional concerns about the grandmother hypothesis.

Finally, menopause can be considered to be adaptive within contemporary, industrialized society. Constant ovulatory cycles, without breaks for multiple pregnancies and lactation, is a recent human condition (Eaton et al. 1994; Eaton and Eaton 1999; Harrell 1977; Strassman 1996). Various lines of evidence suggest that increasing exposure to periodic elevations in levels of estrogen over the reproductive span is related to an increased risk of breast cancer (Kelsey, Gammon, and John 1993). Although menopause may have been adaptive under past conditions by curtailing childbearing so that women were free to invest in the well-being of children and grandchildren, more recent conditions suggest that menopause is also adaptive as an end to breast and other estrogenically sensitive tissue exposure to high, cyclic levels of estrogen. This argument is, however, a difficult one to make without invoking the grandmother hypothesis, since natural selection would otherwise have little reason to favor postreproductive life.

With this argument, menopause lowers the risk of breast cancer, which can strike well before the end of the fertile period and hence directly reduce reproductive success. As Hall (2004) points out, the result of oocyte deterioration and related increases in early fetal losses (miscarriages) is that "older females would be expected to have *more* rather than fewer menstruations" (86, emphasis added). Without the cessation of ovulatory cycles at menopause, women would continue to be exposed to high, cyclic levels of estrogen into the seventh or eighth decade of life. More specifically, their estrogen-receptive target tissues would continue to be exposed to high, cyclic levels of estrogen. In the context of the early menarche, delayed childbirth, and low parity patterns of contemporary Western societies, the cessation of menstrual cycles is adaptive.

Neutral Scenarios for the Evolution of Human Menopause

In most vertebrate species the upper limits of the lifespan correlate with the function of the gonads (Comfort 1979). Humans, short-finned pilot whales (*Globicephala macrorhynchus*), possibly other whales (Marsh and Kasuya 1986), and African elephants (Austad 1997; Finch 1990:165–166) are exceptional in their display of a species-universal post-reproductive period. The chimpanzee, with an maximum lifespan potential of about fifty years, seldom outlives its reproductive function (Graham 1979; Nishida, Takasaki, and Takahata 1990; Nishida et al. 2003). The ability of humans, whales, and possibly elephants to live well beyond a reproductive span supports the hypothesis that there is a phylogenetic constraint of approximately fifty years on oocyte viability among species that finish oogenesis during the fetal period (Pavelka and Fedigan 1991).

It is possible that female hominids were originally fertile to the end of the lifespan, but then the human maximum lifespan potential extended—perhaps through the progressive prolongation of life stages in relation to enlarged brain size or through improved survival at younger ages (Bogin and Smith 1996; Cutler 1976; Hrdy 1999; Lovejoy 1981; Sacher 1978). Maximum lifespan potential represents "the length of life possible for a given species under optimum nutritional and minimal environmental hazard conditions" (Cutler 1978:463). The maximum lifespan potential more than doubled, from the 50-year maximum for chimpanzees to more than 110 years for humans; however, ovarian characteristics such as oocyte number and rate of atresia did not change to the same extent. Menopause, the cessation of menses, was "uncovered" by the extension of the human lifespan. In this scenario the appearance of menopause is architectural (Gould and Lewontin 1979), meaning that menopause is simply a piece of the whole, shaped in part by all of the other pieces.

When, in hominid evolution, did menopause first appear? Fossil evidence suggests that even the more recent bipedal hominids did not live very long (Caspari and Lee 2004). What we cannot tell, from the reconstruction of hominid life tables, is the maximum lifespan potential. Did the shortness of life characteristic of fossil hominids result from reaching the maximum lifespan potential for the species, or did the short life represent the average lifespan possible under PlioPleiostocene conditions?

Indirect evidence offers a glimpse of an answer. Both cranial capacity and body mass measurements used to reconstruct lifespan patterns in fossil humans estimate a maximum lifespan potential of more than fifty years in *Homo erectus* (Bogin and Smith 1996; O'Connell, Hawkes, and Blurton Jones 1999; B. H. Smith 1991). Menopause is, potentially, a very old trait. However, maximum lifespan potential does not necessarily reflect life expectancy. Although *H. erectus* possessed a lengthy lifespan potential, this species of hominid did not leave evidence of the long average lifespan (life expectancy) necessary for the experience of menopause (Caspari and Lee 2004). In other words, as is true for ourselves, menopause was possible for *H. erectus* only if individuals lived long enough.

In another attempt to explain the evolution of menopause and postreproductive life from a nonadaptive point of view, some investigators have focused not on the increase in maximum lifespan potential but on improvement in reaching a higher average life expectancy. Life expectancy is a population-level measure affected by infant mortality and environmental constraints. Wood, Holman, and O'Connor (2001) suggest that menopause can be explained with the concept of antagonistic pleiotropy. Pleiotropy describes how one gene may have multiple effects within the body. In antagonistic pleiotropy, a trait that may be favorable and selected for at early ages (for example, the maintenance of regular cycles at early adult ages through the development of many ovarian follicles) becomes deleterious at later ages (as when older women run out of the ovarian follicles needed to maintain fertile cycles). Wood and colleagues (2001) go on to propose that improved survival at earlier ages enables more individuals to survive to later ages of the lifespan. They write, "post-reproductive life in human females is not adaptive in itself but is an artifact of processes acting at earlier ages. Survival to, say, age seventy involves survival to every age preceding that point. Any evolutionary or cultural change that favors survival to some earlier age, say fifty, will *mutatis mutandis* favor survival to seventy" (486). When women survive to the age of seventy, menopause is "uncovered." Again, menopause is simply a piece of the whole, shaped by all the other parts of the human female lifespan.

CHAPTER THREE

Methods of Study

Itayme Sālem . . . separated her husband from her bed when he took a second wife. 'Alya told us about her. . . . She said to him: I excuse thee concerning the bed and may thy bed be separated from me! Here thou hast one who is fruitful and will bear thee children. I have no longer menstruation and cannot bear either a girl or a boy. I have eaten my share of thee and thou hast eaten thy share of me. Set me free [as if she were a slave] before God's face. I have eaten my fruit and my legs are now crooked.

H. N. Granqvist, *Marriage Conditions in a Palestinian Village* (1935)

After violent storms there will follow a time of intense heat and drought. They say that this is what can be expected of women who are in the stage of life when they cannot bear any more children. "They look back at what was, seeing their sons and their daughters growing up. Then they remember the pains when giving birth and also the sweetness of the children. They remember this and desire very much to give birth again. The heat in them becomes fearful. But their striving for children does not help. The time is past. So it is with this thunder which we say is like women. We say that it is like a woman because it makes much noise and shows great heat, but it brings no rain."

A.-I. Berglund, *Zulu Thought-Patterns and Symbolism* (1976)

As the first epigraph indicates, the topic of menopause is not new to anthropology. Hilma Granqvist carried out fieldwork for her ethnography *Marriage Conditions in a Palestinian Village* (1935) from 1925 to 1927. She described this work as an "excavation of all the customs, habits and ways of thinking" in that one village (Granqvist 1931:4). Since the early twentieth century, cultural or social anthropologists have gathered information on the topic of menopause as part of their ethnographic studies of non-Western peoples.

A perusal of data organized within the Human Relations Area Files (HRAF) demonstrates that early observers of menopause (Cohen 1952; Gladwin and Sarason 1953; Junod 1927; Morris 1938) were primarily interested in whether postmenopausal women remained sexually active (a question that persists in the biomedical literature today).[1] Later observers (Altorki 1986; Bart 1969, 1971; J. Brown 1982; De Young 1955; H. K. Henderson 1969; H. K. Kaufman 1960; Ottenberg 1958; Reynolds 1978; Terwiel 1975) were interested in how women's social roles changed with the shift to postreproductive life. Other anthropologists analyzed symbolic meanings of the cessation of menstruation (Berglund 1976; Buckley and Gottlieb 1988) or focused on the experience of symptoms during the menopause transition (Davis 1986; Lock 1993; E. Martin 1987).

The second epigraph illustrates the study of menopause from a symbolic perspective. We can make an educated guess that the Zulu women studied were experiencing hot flashes ("the heat in them"). Axel-Ivar Berglund, a South African anthropologist and missionary who studied menopause among the Zulu as part of his larger work on the patterns and symbolism of Zulu thought (1976), was interested in the symbolism, not the symptoms, of the menopause transition.[2] In contrast, a biocultural perspective explores both the physical experience and the meaning of menopause. This chapter reviews menopause as a topic of study based in the general population (rather than as a phenomenon in need of medical intervention).

Talking about Menopause

When I carried out my first study of menopause in upstate New York in 1989–1990, I was somewhat surprised by the difficulty I encountered when seeking permission from school superintendents and group leaders to interview women of menopausal age. Hormone therapy (HT) was often in the news and there were frequent ads on television for HT ("Don't let the change of life change yours," coupled with ominous music in the background). Nevertheless, one male superintendent initially refused permission and explained that he didn't want the male teachers and staff to be made uncomfortable. A school nurse intervened and said that she would be sure that the male teachers and staff would not find out about the study. So we surreptitiously handed out fliers to female teachers, bus drivers, cafeteria workers, and custodial staff. The women themselves were happy to talk about menopause—at length.

I also received permission to interview women at a garden club meeting. When I arrived, I found that a large group of older women had gathered to hear a male guest speaker. Several women asked me, in a whisper, not to mention the purpose of my visit until the man left the meeting. So I waited, and they waited, until the man gave his presentation, enjoyed refreshments, and left. Then we talked about menopause.

For a study of menopause in the city of Puebla, Mexico, in 1999–2000, we quickly abandoned a door-to-door method of random sampling and instead recruited an opportunity sample from public parks and markets. The door-to-door method did not yield a single woman who would agree to talk about menopause. However, women easily agreed to be interviewed on the street, often in the company of their friends. They spoke openly about menopause—again, at length.

In contrast, menopause was not an appropriate topic of conversation in Slovenia. During the summer of 2002, at the invitation of Maruška Vidovič, I learned about menopause in the rural, alpine Selška Valley. Here study participants preferred to answer our questions in the privacy of their homes. We learned that women seldom discuss menopause with each other or with their husbands. At the end of the structured interview, respondents visibly relaxed (and brought out their homemade schnapps and cookies).

These details are a reminder that menopause has been, and continues to be, a topic that is uncomfortable for many people. That discomfort influences participant recruitment and hence the results that have been collected over the years.

It is also important to remember that the experience of menopause in one country is not necessarily representative of how menopause is viewed or experienced in other countries. What is meant by "menopause in the United States" or "menopause in Mexico" may not even be representative of the menopausal experience for all populations or subcultures within that one country. For example, much of what we understand about the "normal menopause transition" in the United States comes from longitudinal research carried out among primarily white women from Minnesota (Mansfield and Bracken 2003; Treloar 1974, 1981; Treloar et al. 1967; Whelan et al. 1990) and Massachusetts (Avis, Crawford, and McKinlay 1997; Brambilla and McKinlay 1989; McKinlay, Brambilla, and Posner 1992). Only recently has a four-year cohort study of menopause enrolled equal numbers of African American and white women (Freeman et al. 2001; Grisso et al. 1999). In addition, a large, rigorously designed, longitudinal Study of Women's Health Across the Nation (SWAN) is under way to examine the experience of menopause among women of African, Hispanic, Japanese, Chinese, and European heritage (Avis et al. 2001; Gold et al. 2000; Sowers et al. 2000). The following multidisciplinary review of pioneering work in the study of menopause is not exhaustive, but includes a group of studies selected to illustrate methodological details.

Alan Treloar

The first nonmedical study of menopause in the United States was begun in 1934 by Alan E. Treloar at the University of Minnesota with the help of Ruth Boynton, a physician at the University of Minnesota's Health Service, and Esther Doerr, a master's student (Mansfield and Bracken 2003). Between 1935 and 1939, 2,350 female students were recruited via their entrance health examinations. These students provided their age at menarche and filled out calendar cards documenting their menstrual bleeding over the following decades. Additional

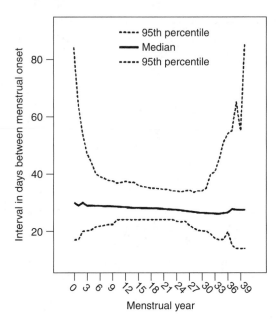

FIGURE 3.1 Variability of menstrual cycle length.

Redrawn from Treloar et al. (1967).

cohorts of women were recruited from other sites, as were daughters and grand-daughters of the original cohort (Mansfield and Bracken 2003; Whelan et al. 1990). Women continued filling out calendar cards year after year. In 1981 Treloar was able to publish results from "763 cases whose menstrual records have terminated in menopause, either natural or surgical, at a precisely recorded date" (249).

Treloar's conscientious research showed, first of all, that the "normal" twenty-eight-day cycle was a myth (Treloar et al. 1967). In fact, the length of the menstrual cycle is quite variable, as shown in figure 3.1, particularly during the years right after menarche (menstrual years 0–5) and the years just prior to menopause (menstrual years 30–39). His data also showed that the average age of menopause among this population of women was 49.5, although the range in ages at menopause stretched from 37 to 56 (Treloar 1974).[3]

Treloar's study was important because it was prospective and longitudinal: it collected multiple measurements for each woman across time. Treloar thus did not have to rely on women's memories for their age at menopause (as in retrospective studies), and he followed them through their entire menstrual career. The study was also important because during the years that Treloar's college coeds were approaching menopause, there were few nonmedical studies of menopause under way. In the same way that individual women must learn to recognize their own menopause, social scientists also had to learn to recognize that menopause was a phenomenon worthy of study.[4]

Treloar's longitudinal study has had a variety of names, but is now called the Tremin Research Program on Women's Health (Tremin comes from "Tre" for Treloar and "Min" for Minnesota). Following Treloar's tenure, the data set was maintained by Anne Voda at the University of Utah (Voda 1997) and now continues under the directorship of Phyllis K. Mansfield at Pennsylvania State University. Presently 1,210 women whose ages range from the early teens to the midnineties are active record keepers (Mansfield and Bracken 2003; www.pop. psu.edu/tremin).

Cross-sectional Studies of the 1960s

In the Netherlands, a large cross-sectional study of age at menopause was carried out in 1967. Unlike longitudinal studies, cross-sectional studies take one measurement at one point in time from many participants. Laszlo Jaszmann and colleagues (1969) spent two years preparing the community of Ede through lectures at women's clubs and a publicity campaign in local newspapers. Only then did researchers send questionnaires to 6,628 women, aged forty-two to sixty-two, living in the borough. The number of forms returned was 4,584 (a 71 percent response rate). Results included the findings that the median age of menopause was 51.4 years (±3.8 years) (Jaszmann, van Lith, and Zaat 1969), and women in their early postmenopausal years complained more frequently of hot flashes, sweats, and pains in muscles and joints than did women in the initial stages of the menopause transition (Jaszmann 1973). Malcolm Whitehead makes the additional point that Jaszmann was one of the first to suggest that certain psychological symptoms might be related to changes in ovarian status, "and we have spent much of the last twenty years trying to confirm or refute this link" (Whitehead 1994:4).[5]

This early study in Ede illustrates some characteristics of good menopause studies that are still valid. First, menopause was defined as the last menstrual period followed by twelve months of amenorrhea. This is still the definition of menopause most widely used and the definition recommended by the World Health Organization (1981, 1996). Second, probit analysis was used to compute a median age at menopause (the point at which half of the women in the population were still menstruating and half of the women had experienced menopause). Figure 3.2 shows the results of a probit analysis computed by Susan Hautaniemi Leonard using data from Puebla, Mexico.

Probit analysis and life table techniques are the best methods in use to determine age at menopause for any population (discussed in more detail in Chapter Four). Finally, Jaszmann and colleagues (1969) separated women into two groups: those who experienced menopause by hysterectomy and those who experienced a natural menopause. Studies of age at menopause still exclude women who undergo menopause by hysterectomy (unless hysterectomies are included as

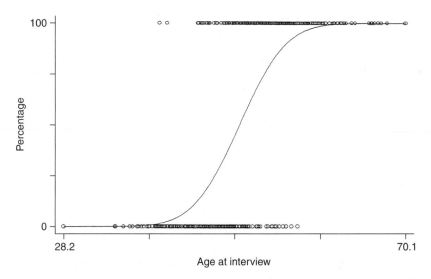

FIGURE 3.2 Probit analysis was used to compute the median age at menopause in Puebla, Mexico. The open circles along the bottom of the graph indicate premenopausal women. The oldest premenopausal woman is fifty-six. The open circles along the top of the graph indicate naturally postmenopausal women. Two women are postmenopausal by age thirty. The curved line indicates the estimated percentage of women who are postmenopausal at each year of age. The median age at menopause is the point at which 50 percent of the women are still menstruating and 50 percent of the women are postmenopausal. That point is found at age 49.6 years.

Courtesy of Susan Hautaniemi Leonard.

censored observations in life table analyses). The 1967 study in Ede was repeated in 1977 (Brand and Lehert 1978) and again in 1987 (Oldenhave and Jaszmann 1991; Oldenhave et al. 1993), allowing researchers to test for a secular trend in age at menopause over time. A secular trend is a change in a characteristic within a population over time, such as an increase in height or a decrease in age at menarche. Some have argued that over time, menopause occurs at later ages (Rodstrom et al. 2003). Most researchers disagree (Flint 1997; Peccei 1999).

Another early cross-sectional study of age at menopause was carried out by MacMahon and Worcester (1966) for the United States Department of Health, Education, and Welfare. In this study, average age at menopause was computed by a method similar to probit analysis to be 49.8 years among 1,315 women ages forty to sixty. Although both cross-sectional studies were carried out in the 1960s, one striking difference between the Netherlands study and the U.S. study was the high number of women who had undergone a hysterectomy in the United States (22 percent) compared with the low rate of hysterectomies (6 percent) in the sample drawn from Ede. The United States continues to have one of the highest hysterectomy rates in the world, so that by age sixty, 37 percent of all U.S. women have undergone the procedure (Pokras and Hufnagel 1988). Rates for hysterectomy in 1990 were 5.5 per 1,000 women, with an increase to 5.6 per 1,000 women by 1997 (Farquhar and Steiner 2002). Factors that put women at risk of hysterectomies are discussed in more detail at the end of this chapter.

To recap the studies above, average age at menopause in the United States and northern Europe, during the 1960s and 1970s, was forty-nine to fifty-one years. This continues to be the median age at menopause in the United States and Europe today. When did social scientists in the United States recognize symptoms associated with menopause as an engaging area of study? This also began during the 1960s and 1970s, initially with the work of the sociologist Bernice Neugarten in Chicago.

Bernice Neugarten

Described as a sociologist's psychologist and a psychologist's sociologist (Hagestad 1996), Bernice Neugarten enjoyed a professional career that spanned fifty years. We drew on her work earlier, in Chapter One, when we applied concepts related to the lifespan approach, such as "on time" and "off time" (Neugarten and Datan 1973) and "age norms or age expectations" (Neugarten 1969). In an autobiographical piece, Neugarten (1996) commented that the "unpredicted turn of events in my own career [that led to the study of aging] may be one of the reasons for my belief that, in the study of human lives, insufficient attention has been given to the unanticipated and the off-time events, to the discontinuities as well as the continuities" (6). Her thoughts have obvious application to the study of menopause as an event within the lifespan.

In 1963 Neugarten et al. published the first study of women's attitudes toward menopause. Attitudes were measured by a series of statements with which women were asked to agree or disagree. (Examples of the questions are given in table 6.4.) Central to their findings was the realization that younger women had more fears about menopause than middle-aged and older women. The finding that premenopausal women have more fears about menopause compared with postmenopausal women has been repeated across cultures (Sievert and Espinosa-Hernández 2003).

Shortly after this study of attitudes, Neugarten and Kraines (1965) published a study of menopausal symptoms that compared complaints reported by menopausal women with those reported by women of other ages (ages thirteen to sixty-four, $n = 460$). Neugarten and Kraines developed their symptom checklist from the medical literature and from preliminary interviews and characterized twelve symptoms as somatic (for example, hot flashes, rheumatic pains), eleven as psychological (for example, irritability and nervousness, feeling blue), and five as psychosomatic (for example, pounding of the heart, headaches). They found that somatic and psychosomatic symptoms were reported most often by menopausal women. In contrast, adolescents reported the greatest number of psychological symptoms. Although the categories of symptoms differed, the increased reporting of complaints at adolescence and at menopause led the study authors to reflect on the social and endocrine similarities between adolescence and the menopause transition. They noted that "it is the increased production of sex hormones during adolescence (signaled by the first menses) and the decreased production of estrogen during the climacterium (signaled by menopause) that are primary in producing heightened sensitivity to and an increased frequency of reported symptoms" (Neugarten and Kraines 1965:272).

Finally, in "The Middle Years," Bernice Neugarten and Nancy Datan (1974) addressed the "unbalanced views" of psychologists who were treating menopause as a crisis. From a social psychological perspective, Neugarten and Datan argued that women in the United States minimized the significance of menopause. They proposed that women welcomed menopause as relief from menstruation and the fear of unwanted pregnancies. This point of view downplayed the understanding of menopause as a hormonal deficiency syndrome, a characterization that was popular in medicine at the time. Neugarten and Datan's efforts to de-medicalize menopause have been continued by many social scientists since then (Bell 1987; Kaufert 1988; Kaufert and Gilbert 1986; Kaufert and Lock 1997; Komesaroff, Rothfield, and Daly 1997; Lock 1993; Macpherson 1985; McCrea 1983; Voda 1997; Worcester and Whatley 1992).

New Beginnings: 1980s and Beyond

In the 1980s menopause became fully recognized as a topic of study within the social sciences. One of the most important developments was a trio of studies carried out in Massachusetts, Canada, and Japan by investigators who worked together to make their results comparable (Avis et al. 1993; Kaufert et al. 1986; Lock 1998; McKinlay, Brambilla, and Posner 1992). In particular, these investigators rejected symptom lists developed by medical practitioners in the 1950s, such as the Kupperman/Blatt Menopausal Index, in favor of a symptom list that embedded discomforts associated with menopause within a catalog of Everyday Complaints (for example, coughs and stomachaches).

In 1981–82 the epidemiologist Sonya McKinlay and colleagues began a prospective, longitudinal study of menopause in Massachusetts. At that time, McKinlay was already established as a menopause researcher in Great Britain (McKinlay, Jefferys, and Thompson 1972; McKinlay and Jefferys 1974). She and her husband, John McKinlay, had published one of the earliest critiques of menopause studies (McKinlay and McKinlay 1973), which influenced and improved all of the studies that followed. In that critique, the McKinlays lamented "a general lack of interest in providing comparable or consistent data" (534) in the study of menopause. They argued for a consistent and relatively objective definition of menopause, for agreement on the symptoms that made up a "menopausal syndrome," and for improved sampling of healthy women who were going to experience a natural menopause. Instead of relying on medical discussions of symptomatology "usually with no clear empirical basis" (535), the transition to menopause should be studied among one or more cohorts of women, sampled from healthy populations, and followed prospectively over a period years.

Compared with Treloar's work in Minnesota, the Massachusetts Women's Health Study was of short duration—only five years in length. McKinlay and her colleagues, however, interviewed many more women as they approached and passed through the menopause transition. The initial random sample, collected from town and city census lists, yielded 2,565 participants aged forty-five to fifty-five. Participants were women who had menstruated in the three months prior to the survey and had agreed to answer six telephone interviews carried out at nine-month intervals from 1982 to 1987 (Brambilla and McKinlay 1989; McKinlay, Brambilla, and Posner 1992). Median age at menopause was 51.3 years. The perimenopause (defined as a change in cycle regularity in at least two consecutive interviews and/or three to eleven months of amenorrhea) began almost four years earlier, at a median age of 47.5 (McKinlay, Brambilla, and Posner 1992). Women with more negative attitudes toward menopause prior to the experience were more likely to report hot flashes at menopause (Avis, Crawford, and McKinlay 1997).

For years, the results of the Massachusetts study served as the model for the "normal" menopause transition, in part because only 1.9 percent of the 2,570 participants were using any sort of hormone therapy when the longitudinal study began in the early 1980s (McKinlay, Brambilla, and Posner 1992). HT use, which can dampen hot flashes and cause continued menstrual cycles, reached frequencies of 60 percent or higher in some cities in the United States in the early 1990s (Von Mühlen, Kritz-Silverstein, and Barrett-Conner 1995). More details about the rise, fall, rise, and fall of HT use in the United States are given in Chapter Six.

In Canada, the sociologist Patricia Kaufert and colleagues carried out a study of midlife and menopause entitled the Manitoba Project on Women and Their Health. First, a survey was mailed to 2,500 women, aged forty to fifty-nine, who were selected from the general population of women in the province of Manitoba. The response rate was 68 percent. Following the cross-sectional survey, a longitudinal study was carried out for three years among women who were forty-five years of age or older and who had either menstruated within the past three months ($n = 369$) or had previously had a hysterectomy ($n = 136$). Interviews every six months were taken by telephone. Findings included the demonstration that twelve months without menstruation is generally long enough to establish that menopause has occurred (Kaufert, Gilbert, and Tate 1987) and that natural menopause does not increase the odds that a woman will become depressed (Kaufert, Gilbert, and Tate 1992).

In Japan, the cultural anthropologist Margaret Lock combined survey and interview methods to better understand kōnenki, best translated to mean the change of life. In 1984 a survey was distributed in the prefectures of Kobe, Kyoto, and Nagano to 1,738 women aged forty-five to fifty-five. Women were drawn from a city hall register (Kobe), factories, women's organizations, and forestry and fishing villages. According to Lock, the survey tried "to minimize the impact of preconceived notions" by beginning with a long list of questions about general health and reproductive history. "Explicit inquiries about kōnenki occur only when women are already halfway through their responses" (Lock 1993:31). Of the 1,316 women who filled out the questionnaire, 105 participants agreed to a semi-structured and open-ended interview. Most interviews took place in the women's homes.

Lock's book *Encounters with Aging: Mythologies of Menopause in Japan and North America* (1993) illustrates the unique experience of individual women as they went through the ambiguous change of life, a transition not necessarily associated with the end of menstruation in Japan as it is in the United States. This detailed examination of aging in Japan offers a basis for reflexive objectivity, a chance to look back at the United States with more clarity to see how the medicalization of women's aging is a cultural peculiarity, rather than a biological necessity.

In addition to the three studies carried out in Massachusetts, Canada, and Japan, the Australian researcher Lorraine Dennerstein applied similar methods and the same symptom list in the Melbourne Women's Midlife Health Project in 1991. Her aims were to describe women's symptom experience during the natural menopause transition and to investigate the relative contributions of menopause, health status, social factors, and lifestyle behaviors to midlife symptoms (http://www.psychiatry.unimelb.edu.au/midlife/). For the cross-sectional survey, women aged forty-five to fifty-five were recruited from the Melbourne metropolitan area by means of randomly selected telephone numbers. From 54,078 phone calls, 2,001 women were found to be eligible and available for the study (Smith et al. 1992). These women completed a 20–25 minute telephone interview (Dennerstein et al. 1993). Among the results were the reassuring findings that these midlife women felt clear-headed (72 percent), good-natured (71 percent), useful (68 percent), satisfied (61 percent), understood (60 percent), confident (58 percent), and loving (56 percent) most of the time (Dennerstein 1994).

Of the initial 2,001 women, 438 agreed to continue in a seven-year longitudinal study. Women in the longitudinal study had menstruated in the three months prior to the first interview and were not taking oral contraceptives or HT. Once each year, follow-up questionnaires were given and physical measures were collected in women's homes. In contrast to the exclusive use of surveys in Massachusetts, Canada, and Japan, Dennerstein worked with endocrinologist Henry Burger to monitor blood levels of FSH, estradiol, inhibin and other hormones across the menopause transition (Burger et al. 1995, 1998, 1999, 2002).

On an annual basis, follicle stimulating hormone and estradiol were assayed from blood samples collected between days four and eight of the menstrual cycle, or after three months of amenorrhea. Maximum change in levels of FSH and E2 occurred during the late perimenopause, defined as having had three to eleven months of amenorrhea (Dennerstein et al. 2000).

The studies carried out in Massachusetts, Canada, Japan, and Australia have made important methodological contributions, including the use of strictly random community-based samples from a general population, objective definitions of menopause stages, and the use of comparable, validated, and reliable instruments (Dennerstein 1996). A validated instrument is one which accurately measures what it aims to measure, regardless of who participates in the study, when she participates, and who asks the questions. A reliable instrument measures the same results in the same way, each time it is used.

Table 3.1 summarizes some symptom frequencies collected across the four studies. The results are comparable because the question pertaining to symptom frequencies was asked in the same way (during the past two weeks, have you experienced . . .?) using very similar symptom lists. Difficulties associated with the translation of this list for the Japanese are discussed later in this chapter.

As in Melbourne, both social and biological data were collected in the Seattle Midlife Women's Health Study. In Seattle, the original population-based

TABLE 3.1

The Percentage of Women of Menopausal Age Who Reported Symptoms during the Two Weeks before Interview

Symptom	Massachusetts	Canada	Japan	Australia
Hot flashes	35	31	12	32
Cold sweats	11	20	4	10
Nervousness or irritability	30	17	12	41
Feeling blue or depressed	36	23	10	33
Headache	37	34	28	36
Back pain	30	27	24	38

Sources: Massachusetts, Canada, and Japan: Lock (1998); Australia: Dennerstein et al. (1993).

Note: The four studies used similar recruitment techniques and methodologies.

sample was obtained in 1990–1992 by a telephone screening of 11,222 households within census tracts selected for mixed ethnicity and income. Of the 820 women who met the eligibility criteria, 508 women aged thirty-five to fifty-five enrolled in the study. The eligibility criteria included having one or both ovaries intact, having had at least one menstrual period in the previous twelve months, and being able to read and understand English (Mitchell, Woods, and Mariella 2000). In addition to answering questions about symptoms associated with midlife, women were asked to keep daily health diaries and yearly menstrual calendars and, between 1997 and 2000, urine specimens were collected once a month to assay FSH, estrone, and cortisol levels (Mitchell, Woods, and Mariella 2003; Woods, Mitchell, and Mariella 2003). Estrone is a form of estrogen. Cortisol is a hormone secreted by the adrenal glands in response to physical or psychological stress.

Finally, at this writing a large multiethnic, multisite study is being carried out to examine quality of life, disease risk, and symptoms at midlife across the United States (Avis et al. 2003; Bromberger et al. 2004; Matthews et al. 2005). This Study of Women's Health Across the Nation began with a cross-sectional telephone or in-home survey in 1995–1997, and continues as a longitudinal investigation tracking health changes as women go through the menopause transition. The seven locations in which the study is being carried out are Boston; Chicago; Detroit; Los Angeles; Newark, NJ; Oakland, CA; and Pittsburgh. At the start of the study, all seven sites sampled white women. African Americans were sampled in Pittsburgh, Boston, Detroit, and Chicago. Women of Japanese heritage were sampled in Los Angeles, of Chinese heritage in Oakland, and of Hispanic heritage in Newark. Community-based sampling was possible for all samples at five sites, but a "snowball" approach was required at the two sites with Hispanic and Japanese samples (Avis et al. 2001; Gold et al. 2000; Sowers et al. 2000).[6]

These studies carried out in the United States, Canada, Japan, and Australia are recognized as large, well-designed, authoritative studies of the menopause transition. Excellent studies have also been carried out in Finland (Hemminki, Topo, and Kangas 1995; Luoto, Kaprio, and Uutela 1994), Holland (den Tonkelaar, Seidell, and van Noord 1996; van Noord et al. 1997), Norway (Holte 1992), England (Hardy and Kuh 2002a, 2005; M. S. Hunter 1990; Kuh et al. 1997, 2002), and elsewhere in the United States (Wilbur et al. 1998).

Cross-Cultural Comparisons

Alongside the large longitudinal studies sits a collection of smaller cross-sectional studies, many of which have been carried out in non-Western countries. These smaller surveys offer cross-cultural data for comparison and uncover aspects of human variation associated with menopause that larger, systematic surveys sometimes miss. Some of the first, and arguably the most important, work of this type was that of Marcha Flint. Malcolm Whitehead noted, in a tribute to menopause researcher Pieter van Keep, that he knew van Keep "was impressed by Marcha Flint's early work which reported that Rajput Indians did not experience hot flushes at menopause. Clearly there were many cross-cultural differences which at that time were waiting to be identified and elucidated" (Whitehead 1994:3).[7] As Whitehead implies, Flint's work inspired a generation of research.

Flint, a biological anthropologist, studied menopause in India as part of her City University of New York dissertation "Menarche and Menopause of Rajput Women" (1974). She surveyed 483 women of the Rajput caste in the states of Rajasthan and Himachal Pradesh and concluded that very few women had any problems with their menopause. "There were no depressions, dizziness, no incapacitations nor any of the symptoms associated with what we call 'the menopausal syndrome'" (Flint 1975:162). Flint carried out her research during a time when women's social roles were emphasized, and her interpretations were consistent with this emphasis: "In Rajasthan, Rajput women who, until their menopause, had to live in *purdah* (veiled and secluded) could now come downstairs from their women's quarters to where the men talked and drank their home brew. . . . In Himachal Pradesh, the Rajput women could publicly visit and joke with men after attaining menopause. These women were no longer considered to be contaminative" (162). She argued that these women experienced no symptoms with the menopause transition because menopause was associated with positive role changes.

Flint motivated further research when she published a brief article in *Psychosomatics,* the official journal of the Academy of Psychosomatic Medicine. The paper began with a detailed review of the biology of menopause and hot flashes. In the middle of the second page, Flint described her study findings. She then presented a short review of the anthropological literature, and ended with the clinical relevance of her findings. In three pages, Flint crossed the boundary between social science and biomedicine and communicated that in India women do not have hot flashes and "that much of what we call 'menopausal symptomatology' may well be culturally defined" (163). Vatuk (1975) corroborated these findings, but it was Flint who disseminated them to a multidisciplinary audience. Later Margaret Lock demonstrated the same skill in communicating cross-cultural evidence across the social scientific/biomedical boundary (1991, 1998).

Another early, influential study was carried out by Dona Lee Davis in 1977–1978 in Grey Rock Harbour, a Newfoundland fishing village (Davis 1983). She found that Newfoundland women viewed menopause as a social/personal problem rather than as a biomedical issue. Her conclusions, based on thirty-eight interviews, placed the experience of menopause squarely within the context of being a fisherman's wife—a life of worry, responsibility, and, at the same time, relatively high female status. In addition, Davis emphasized the culturally specific concepts of "blood" and "nerves" that were used to describe or explain health. For example, "at menopause blood can 'go up.' Women who have hysterectomies are particularly prone to high blood because 'all the blood has nowhere to go'" (135). "Nerves" were the most common complaint given by middle-aged women besides hot flashes, which could also be called "nervous flashes." Other problems attributed to "the change" included loss of patience, forgetfulness, tiredness, and lack of judgment. Davis learned that women just "aren't the same anymore" (141), and strong female networks provided support for those who experienced difficulty.

Another study that inspired a great deal of interest in menopause across cultures was carried out by Yewoubdar Beyene. Beyene (1989) contrasted the experience of menopause in two farming communities, Stira, Greece, and Chichimilá, Yucatán, Mexico. It was her work in Yucatán that attracted the most attention, because, like Flint, Beyene reported an absence of hot flashes. According to Beyene, Maya women perceived menopause to be an event that occurs when a woman has used up all of her menstrual blood. Menopause was simply called the time when menstrual periods completely stop, "cuando se acaba la regla por completo" (Beyene 1989:119). In contrast to Flint's findings in India, menopause for Maya women was not associated with positive (or negative) changes in household roles. Nevertheless, similar to Flint's findings, no Maya women described the experience of hot flashes (Beyene 1986, 1989; Martin et al. 1993). Because Beyene lived within the Chichimilá community for a year, she was convinced that the lack of hot flashes was a real finding and not the result of an inappropriate translation.

Other small studies have established that while the average age at menopause hovers around fifty in developed countries, the mean age at menopause in developing countries can be much younger. For example, among the Agta of Cagayan Province, Philippines, Goodman et al. (1985) found that menopause was experienced as never getting a period following one's last childbirth. Mean age of this postpartum menopause was quite early, 43.9 ± 2.37 ($n = 15$), following an average of 6.5 live births. Beyene (1989) reported a similarly early age at menopause among the Maya.

As already mentioned, my own experience in the study of menopause has taken me from upstate New York to western Massachusetts; Puebla, Mexico; the Selška Valley of Slovenia; Paraguay; and Hilo, Hawaii. Throughout this book I draw on details from this fieldwork, primarily from Puebla, to illustrate women's experience with the menopause transition and to detail population variation in age and symptom experience at menopause.

I should note that because of my interest in menopause, my understandings of politics, religion, social relationships, values, and the tasks of everyday life are largely shaped by middle-aged women. I have always lived with middle-aged women in Mexico; I collaborate with middle-aged women in Slovenia;

I have interviewed hundreds of middle-aged women; and now I *am* a middle-aged woman. In defense of this perspective, I can only quote Hilma Granqvist, who said, "Those who have women as informants are in a specially favourable position; the women are very much interested in their conditions and linger with pleasure over things which the men glide over lightly" (1931:22). With this I strongly concur. To put the details drawn from Puebla in context, I focus here on my study carried out from 1999 to 2000.[8]

Puebla is the capital city of the state of Puebla, with a population of more than 1.2 million residents (2000 census). A city known for its Catholic faith, Puebla also offers socioeconomic diversity and a broad range of variation in education levels and access to health care. There is also variation in the extent to which women are aware of, and have access to, the medical management of menopause. In Puebla, women learn about menopause through television programs (for example, *Con Sello de Mujer*, a program for women aired every weekday morning on a popular network station, tvazteca) and advertising (for herbal preparations such as Mensifem and other products),[9] radio programs, public conferences sponsored by private menopause clinics, and magazines such as *Buen Hogar* (Good Housekeeping) and *Selecciones* (Reader's Digest).

My colleagues and I carried out a community study of age and symptom experience at menopause from May 1999 through August 2000. Women (*n* = 755) were recruited from public parks, on the streets outside of their homes, in open markets, in small shops, and in front of large public buildings such as the Social Security hospital. Although women aged forty to sixty were targeted, sometimes it was hard to guess a woman's age, and we didn't want to refuse participation to anyone who wanted to be in the study. Therefore seventeen participants were younger than forty years and thirty-five were older than sixty years of age at the time of interview. Interviews lasted twenty-five to fifty minutes and took place on the spot or at a later appointment. Interviews often took place in the company of friends or extended family members.

Using a detailed street map, the research team met each week to talk about where we had been and where we planned to go. Slowly we canvassed the entire city, neighborhood by neighborhood, in the hopes of achieving representation from all social classes (Sievert and Hautaniemi 2003). In general, mean age at interview was 50.1 years (s.d. 6.3); women reported relatively low levels of education (8.1 years) and had, on average, 3.6 children. Additional sample characteristics are shown in table 3.2.

To make our results comparable with those of other studies, we used the same symptom list used by McKinlay in Massachusetts, Kaufert in Canada, Lock in Japan, and Dennerstein in Australia. We focused on collecting information related to factors suspected to be associated with variation in age at menopause (for example, socioeconomic status and smoking habits) and variation in symptom experience (for example, diet and breastfeeding patterns).

TABLE 3.2

Characteristics of the Community Sample Drawn from Puebla, Mexico
($n = 755$)

Characteristics

Mean age at interview (s.d.)	50.1 (6.3)
Mean years of education (s.d.)	8.1 (4.4)
Speak an indigenous language	3%
Marital status	66% married, 13% single, 11% widowed, 6% divorced, 3% living with male partner
Employed outside of the home	63%
Percentage of smokers	18%
Number of children (s.d.)	3.6 (2.3)
Rate of hysterectomy	23%
Using HT at the time of interview	11.7%

Just as Margaret Lock (1993) learned in Japan, I also found that, in Mexico, *la menopausia* is a unique experience for each woman. Women described menopause as *natural, normal,* as an opportunity to save money spent on menstrual pads, as a time to mature as a woman (*madurar más como mujer*), as synonymous with *freedom* and *la tranquilidad,* as a phase of life ordained by God. Women commonly described menopause as freedom from worries about pregnancy. Relatedly, some said that their sexual relations improved. One fifty-seven-year-old woman, mother of four, said that when life gives you menopause, "Tiene que aceptarlo con amor" (You have to accept it with love). "La gloria de seguir viviendo" (The blessing of continued life), stated a fifty-one-year-old administrative assistant. "Que bello es no volver a reglar jamas!" (How beautiful it is to never have to menstruate again), commented a fifty-four-year-old woman with enthusiasm who, earlier in the interview, described her menstruation as very heavy ("muy abundante").

In contrast to the positive reaction of some, others were more negative, because with menopause they felt worse, weighed more, were worried about symptoms, and lost desire for sexual relations. Many premenopausal women expressed concerns about menopause because they had seen other women go through difficult times. "Ve en otras mujeres que se ponen mal" (You can see how other women become ill), said a forty-two-year-old saleswoman. "Ya no puede tener hijos aunque se siente joven" (You can't have children, even though you feel young) stated a fifty-one-year-old mother of three who said that, with menopause, she cried a lot and experienced anxiety. Other women expressed *preocupación* (worry) because they lacked information about menopause and didn't know what would happen.

Although a great deal of individual variation was evident, it is possible to identify some general differences in menopausal experience between Puebla, Mexico, and Japan (Lock 1993) or Yucatán, Mexico (Beyene 1989). For example, in Puebla, women identified menopause as a life event that is part of, yet separate from, aging. This differs from Lock's conclusions in Japan, where menopause is an ambiguous life event. In Puebla, the urban women were likely to volunteer symptoms that they associated with menopause, particularly hot flashes, and they were likely to worry about menopause as a difficult time. This differs from Beyene's conclusions in the same country, but with a different population; Maya women did not report hot flashes or worry about menopause. Cross-cultural studies broaden our understanding of the menopause transition by showing that age and symptom experience at menopause is an aspect of human variation, like childhood growth (Bogin 1999; Eveleth and Tanner 1990), skin color (Frisancho 1993; Relethford 1997), blood pressure (James and Brown 1997), or nose shape (S. Molnar 2002). Defining the "normal" menopause transition is useful for biomedical concerns; "normal," however, has most often been based on data from Western populations. Anthropology expands the concept of normal by including the rest of the world: new ranges of variation refine our ideas of normality.

Questions and Cohorts

In addition to cross-cultural variation, the findings from one generation may or may not apply to the next (James, Broege, and Schlussel 1996). Factors associated with the menopausal experience vary across age cohorts within the same culture.

A cohort is a group of people who are defined by a particular year, or number of years, of birth (Neugarten and Datan 1973). For example, in her study of menopause in Newfoundland, Davis (1983) details how women's lives were changed by the introduction of a road to the fishing village. The year the road was built became the cutoff for comparing older, traditional female roles with the social roles of younger, contemporary women. As many studies have shown, a woman's sociocultural environment is determined, in part, by cohort membership that shapes economic experience, health behavior, and diet (Brim and Kagan 1980; Elder 1985; Riley 1982). Variation among cohorts necessitates the lifespan approach discussed in Chapter One.

Variables that change across age cohorts within the same culture include diet, activity patterns, smoking habits, and the degree to which menopause is treated as a medical condition. At present, for example, the world is witnessing

an epidemic of obesity. In the United States, almost 65 percent of the adult population is overweight, defined as having a BMI greater than 25 kg/m^2. Thirty-one
percent are obese, defined as having a BMI greater than 30 kg/m^2. If weight gain
continues at the present rate, by 2008, 39 percent of the U.S. population will be
obese (Hill et al. 2003). The WHO estimates that worldwide, in 2000, over 300
million adults were obese, up from 200 million five years before (www.who.int/
nut/obs.htm). This epidemic of obesity must be kept in mind when one consid-
ers changes in symptom frequencies that may be associated with body mass,
such as hot flashes or joint pain, across time.

The mean BMI among women sampled in Puebla was 29.0 kg/m^2 (s.d. 2.3),
similar to the mean BMI of 29.9 kg/m^2 reported in León, Guanajuato, Mexico,
among women of similar age (Huerta et al. 1995). As figure 3.3 shows, 73 percent
of the Puebla sample have a BMI greater than 25 kg/m^2, and 37 percent of the
sample has a BMI greater than 30 kg/m^2. Does the weight gained by women in
Puebla partly explain the higher frequency of hot flashes and "bone pain" experienced within this population? Maybe. This educated guess is based in part on
the observation that heavier women in Puebla report significantly more hot
flashes and joint pain compared with thinner women (Sievert and Goode-Null
2005). In addition, Beyene (1986, 1989) reported a lack of hot flashes among Maya
women in Yucatán. These women are thinner, with a mean BMI of about 26 kg/m^2
(Beyene and Martin 2001; Martin et al. 1993). More evidence for the effect of BMI
on hot flashes is presented in Chapter Six; here we note that the present-day epidemic of obesity may affect changes in symptom rates across time.

Just as diet and activity patterns change across temporal cohorts, so do other
health-related behaviors. In western Massachusetts, for example, a number of

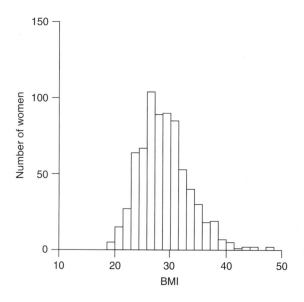

FIGURE 3.3 Range in
BMI among women of
menopausal age,
Puebla, Mexico.

women who are now reaching menopause volunteered that they have been smoking marijuana all their adult lives. This activity was probably less common among women reaching menopause twenty years ago, and it never occurred to me, in 1994, to include marijuana use in a list of questions about health-related behavior among women of menopausal age.

Rodent studies have shown that exposure to marijuana extract (Δ^9-tetrahydrocannabinol, Δ^9-THC) results in a dose-related, transient suppression of LH pulses from the anterior pituitary (Murphy et al. 1998). In ovariectomized rhesus monkeys intramuscular doses of Δ^9-THC cause decreases in both LH and FSH levels (Smith et al. 1979), and when Δ^9-THC is administered during the menstrual cycle, normal estrogen and LH surges and progesterone elevation do not occur (Asch et al. 1981). However, tolerance to the effects of Δ^9-THC appears to develop (Smith et al. 1983) and marijuana has no effect on LH levels in menopausal women (Mendelson et al. 1985). There are cannabinoid receptors in the ovaries, suggesting that the effects of marijuana may occur at the ovary as well as at the pituitary, but the direct ovarian effects are not yet known (Murphy et al. 1998). Whether or not smoking marijuana affects either age at menopause (through an effect on the ovary) or hot flash frequency (through an effect on the hypothalamus, pituitary, or ovary) is an open question. As women who came of age in the 1960s and 1970s are now going through menopause, the question is relevant and should be asked in new or ongoing studies of menopause in the United States.

Cultures, Cohorts, and Methodology

In Japan, it appears that the frequency of hot flashes has been increasing. When Margaret Lock carried out her study of menopause in Japan in 1984, she reported a relatively low frequency of hot flashes (12 percent) among women of menopausal age (Lock 1986, 1993). More recently, hot flash frequencies of 22 percent and higher have been reported in Japan (Anderson et al. 2002; Melby 2005; Nagata et al. 1999; Zeserson 2001). The apparent change in hot flash frequencies within Japan may be related to cohort changes such as increasing Westernization of diet across time, or to broader cultural changes, which include an increasing awareness of menopause as a health-related condition resulting in an increased sensitivity to and labeling of hot flashes (Lock 2005; Zeserson 2001).

The differences may also, however, be the consequence of different sampling techniques and research instruments. For example, Margaret Lock mailed questionnaires to an urban middleclass sample drawn from the register of names and addresses available at Kobe city hall. She also distributed questionnaires to factory workers in Kyoto and obtained a sample of farmworkers through women's organizations in Nagano for a final sample of 1,316 women aged forty-five to fifty-five (Lock 1993:391–392). Melby (2005) recruited 140 women aged forty-five to fifty-five from public health centers, women's groups, parent associations, and women's networks in the Kyoto and Fukushima prefectures. Participants completed an eighty-two-item general health symptoms checklist on their own, between two lengthy interviews. A number of terms were used to describe hot flashes, and all of the terms together measured a hot flash prevalence of 22 percent. Anderson et al. (2002) selected women aged forty-five to sixty from electoral rolls in the Osaka and Nagano regions in Japan. In spite of a sampling strategy that was similar to Lock's, Anderson et al. (2002) found a substantially higher hot flash frequency of 45.3 percent among 1,430 study participants. The subset of 829 participants from Nagano reported a hot flash frequency of 47 percent (Anderson et al. 2004). Nagata et al. (1999) recruited 306 women aged forty to fifty-nine from a health checkup program at a general hospital in Gifu, Japan, and found a hot flash frequency of 37 percent. Zeserson (2001) carried out long interviews in Ehime Prefecture (1992–1993) with 49 women contacted through professional societies and social groups. Of the 44 participants who returned her follow-up questionnaire, 21 participants reported that they had "experienced the feeling of becoming suddenly hot" (201).

With regard to research instruments, Lock and Melby used a symptom checklist that embedded menopausal discomforts into a list of everyday complaints (Avis et al. 1993; Lock 1998; Melby 2005). Anderson et al. (2002, 2004) administered a scale of forty-five items—the MS-45 scale developed by Ysohizawa, Atogami, and Hirasishi. Nagata et al. (1999) used the Blatt/Kupperman index of menopausal distress. Thus although the apparent increase in frequency of hot flashes in Japan over time, from 12 percent to 22 percent or more, may be related to the consumption of an increasingly westernized diet, it may also be due to different sampling strategies, research instruments (symptom lists), or research techniques (mailed questionnaires versus interviews).

Making Cross-Cultural Comparisons

It is difficult to state with certainty that any one variable has a particular effect on any one discomfort associated with the menopause transition. Variables of interest take on culture-specific attributes that lead to multiple caveats in any thorough research report. For example, smoking—a variable often associated with hot flashes—is characteristic of lower socioeconomic levels in the United States, but upper socioeconomic levels in Mexico. In addition, Mexican women of menopausal age tend to smoke five or fewer cigarettes per day while women in their twenties smoke much more heavily. Smoking is common in Lebanon (Obermeyer, Ghorayeb, and Reynolds 1999), but taboo in Nigeria (Okonofua, Lawal, Bamgbose 1990). In addition, smoking may signify tobacco cigarettes to most study participants, but others may include the use of marijuana or a waterpipe (Obermeyer, Ghorayeb, and Reynolds 1999) as smoking behavior. Broad, underlying differences between cultures and age cohorts always need to be kept in mind when one is seeking to explain differences in symptom frequencies within and between cultures or across time. In addition to these concerns, differences in sampling techniques and research questionnaires must also be assessed.

Discomforts associated with menopause are immediately sensitive to health-related behaviors, such as smoking or coffee intake, diet, medical interpretation, or changes in weight-bearing activity. In addition, like age at menopause, discomforts such as hot flashes may also be influenced by events or behaviors associated with earlier points in the lifespan, for example, prepubertal weight gain or attitude formation. Challenging though they may be, cross-cultural and cohort comparisons of symptoms at menopause are valuable for understanding many aspects of women's health and well-being (Avis et al. 1993; Bernis 2001; Beyene 1989; Lock 1993, 1998; Obermeyer 2000; Sievert 2001b).

Many researchers develop their own lists of menopausal discomforts for use in population-specific questionnaires; however, there are three symptom lists that have been repeatedly used in menopause studies: the Blatt/Kupperman Menopausal Index (Blatt, Wiesbader, and Kupperman 1953; Kupperman et al. 1953; Nagata et al. 1999), the Greene Climacteric Scale (Greene 1976, 1998; Holte and Mikkelsen 1991; Hunter, Battersby, and Whitehead 1986), and the list of Everyday Complaints (Avis et al. 1993).

The Blatt/Kupperman Menopausal Index was developed by medical doctors Herbert S. Kupperman and Meyer H. G. Blatt for use in clinical evaluations of the efficacy of estrogenic and nonestrogenic preparations in menopausal and amenorrheic patients (Blatt, Wiesbader, and Kupperman 1953; Kupperman et al. 1953). The Blatt/Kupperman index sought to provide a more objective means of judging and estimating clinical response. Previously, these physicians noted, the criteria for judging the activity of estrogens in the menopausal patient tended "to approach nebulous proportions" (Kupperman et al. 1953:689). Their index permitted a statistical compilation of data to avoid "basing our clinical impression of the different preparations upon 'the shifting sands of empiricism'" (689).

The Blatt/Kupperman index includes eleven menopausal symptoms (table 3.3). The severity of each symptom is scored as 0 (no complaints), 1 (slight), 2 (moderate), or 3 (severe). An index score is calculated by summing up the severity of each symptom multiplied by its weighting factor (Abe et al. 1985; Kupperman et al. 1953; Nagata et al. 1999). Vasomotor symptoms, nervousness, insomnia, and paresthesia (burning or prickling sensations that are usually felt in the extremities) were given more weight in compiling the index because Blatt and colleagues (1953) believed them to be the most important symptoms making up the menopausal syndrome.[10] Table 3.3 gives the original list and a modification of that list as applied in a more recent study in Japan.

Greene (1998) criticized the Blatt/Kupperman Menopausal Index for the way in which it constructed a single score, the total menopausal symptom

TABLE 3.3

**Symptoms Assessed by Two Research Teams Using the
Blatt/Kupperman Menopausal Index**

Kupperman et al.	*Nagata et al.*
Vasomotor complaints	Hot flashes
	Perspiration
	Cold hands and feet
	Shortness of breath
Paresthesia	Tingling of extremities
	Numbness of extremities
Insomnia	Difficulty in getting off to sleep
	Difficulty in staying asleep
Nervousness	Excitable
	Nervous
Melancholia	Feel blue or depressed
Vertigo	Dizziness
Weakness or fatigue	Fatigue
Arthralgia and myalgia	Aches/stiffness in the joints
Headaches	Headache
Palpitation	Palpitations
Formication	Skin-crawling sensations

Source: Kupperman et al. (1953); Nagata et al. (1999).

index. As Greene (1998) pointed out, because the climacteric—the transition from reproductive to nonreproductive life—is "a multifaceted phenomenon, it follows that symptoms occurring during that time may come from different domains, have differing aetiologies and should consequently be categorized and measured separately from each other and not totaled to yield a single score" (26). Instead, Greene chose to review seven factor analyses of menopausal symptoms in order to identify the "facets" of the menopausal syndrome. A factor analysis analyzes the intercorrelations among large numbers of symptoms to identify symptom clusters. "This allows one to delineate the different facets of the symptom picture and to identify those symptoms which are an essential part of the syndrome and those which are not" (Greene 1998:27). Greene

TABLE 3.4

Symptoms Assessed by the Greene Climacteric Scale

Heart beating quickly or strongly	Feeling dizzy or faint
Feeling tense or nervous	Pressure or tightness in head or body
Difficulty in sleeping	Parts of body feeling numb or tingling
Excitable	Headaches
Attacks of panic	Muscle or joint pains
Difficulty in concentrating	Loss of feeling in hands or feet
Feeling tired or lacking in energy	Breathing difficulties
Loss of interest in most things	Hot flushes
Feeling unhappy or depressed	Sweating at night
Crying spells	Loss of interest in sex
Irritability	

Source: Greene (1998).

reviewed factor analyses carried out in Scotland (Greene 1976), India (Indira and Murthy 1980), Canada (Kaufert and Syrotuik 1981), Norway (Holte and Mikkelsen 1991a, b), Japan (Abe et al. 1984), and England (Hunter, Battersby, and Whitehead 1986). He concluded that studies of menopause produce at least three symptom clusters: somatic (including joint pain), psychological (including depression), and vasomotor (including hot flashes).

For his symptom list, Greene chose only symptoms found to have a high factor loading in the original studies. A factor loading is a measure of the relationship between a symptom and the symptom cluster. The resulting Greene Climacteric Scale (shown in table 3.4) has twenty-one symptoms. Sixteen are original to the scale Greene developed in 1976. Women using this scale are to indicate the extent to which they are bothered at the moment by any of the symptoms (not at all, a little, quite a bit, or extremely).

Another response to the Blatt/Kupperman Menopausal Index came from a multidisciplinary group of menopause researchers who met at Korpilampi, Finland, in 1985 to discuss issues related to the definition of menopause, the challenge of cross-cultural research, and the contributions that different disciplines can make to clinical research and practice. Focusing on issues somewhat different from Greene's (1998) concerns, the workshop summary pointed out that simply translating and administering the Blatt/Kupperman symptom list

---

TABLE 3.5

Core Symptoms of the List of Everyday Complaints

Diarrhea/constipation	Dizzy spells
Persistent cough	Lack of energy
Upset stomach	Irritability
Shortness of breath	Feeling blue/depressed
Sore throat	Trouble sleeping
Backaches	Loss of appetite
Headaches	Hot flushes/flashes
Aches/stiffness in joints	Cold or night sweats

Source: Avis et al. (1993).

---

assumes "a universality of symptomology which is probably false and is certainly untested" (Kaufert et al. 1986:1287).

In response to symptom lists that limited researchers to symptoms associated with the Western biomedical model of menopause (see Olazábal Ulacia et al. 1999), members of the Korpilampi workshop developed a list of Everyday Complaints based on a checklist described by Kaufert and Syrotuik (1981). The instrument asks: "Thinking back over the past two weeks, have you been bothered by any of the following?" Table 3.5 shows the sixteen core symptom (Avis et al. 1993).

The Everyday Complaint list minimizes the impact of stereotyping on symptom reports by embedding menopausal symptoms within a list of everyday complaints experienced during the two weeks before interview (Avis et al. 1993). This checklist has now been used across a wide range of populations, allowing for cross-cultural comparisons (Avis et al. 1993; Dennerstein et al. 1993; Hemminki, Topo, and Kangas 1995; Lock 1998; Punyahotra, Dennerstein, and Lehert 1997; Wilbur et al. 1998). The SWAN study described above uses the same format and a subset of the Everyday Complaints checklist (Avis et al. 2001; Gold et al. 2000). I have used the list of Everyday Complaints in western Massachusetts (Leidy 1997; Leidy, Canali, and Callahan 2000); Puebla, Mexico (Sievert 2001a; Sievert and Espinosa-Hernández 2003); and the Selška Valley, Slovenia (Sievert et al. 2004).

Some researchers combine symptom lists, for example, in a study of menopause among women in Beirut, Lebanon, Obermeyer, Ghorayeb, and Reynolds (1999) state that their list of symptoms had a "great deal in common with" the Greene index (Greene 1976, 1998), the list used by the International Health Foundation (Boulet et al. 1994), and the list used in comparative studies of menopause in Massachusetts, Manitoba, and Japan (Avis et al. 1993). Also, like the Menopause Symptom Index (Sarrel and Sarrel 1994), the list used by Obermeyer and colleagues included information on whether or not a symptom occurred occasionally or regularly during the past month, and whether or not this represented a problem. In Paraguay, Mario Carlos González and I used a symptom list based on the Everyday Complaint list and the Greene Climacteric Scale (Sievert et al. 2004).

The use of any survey-type questionnaire depends on informants' understanding the questions and answering them truthfully (Davis 1983). Whether this understanding can be assumed is always a concern when using surveys. Davis expressed other concerns in her work, including the observation that even though particular symptoms make sense to an informant, they may not be considered to be associated with menopause. In addition, symptoms attributed to menopause in a particular cultural context may be absent from checklists. For example, Newfoundland women reported nausea, failing eyesight, and bruises (Davis 1983). In Mexico, I was surprised to find "bone pain" frequently volunteered as a symptom associated with menopause (Sievert and Goode-Null 2005). Finally, Davis cautioned that the explanatory model associated with menopause may vary so dramatically that entire categories of symptoms may vary.

At the very least, symptom checklists need translation, and sometimes additions or deletions, to be culturally appropriate. For example, Obermeyer and colleagues (1999) found that women in pilot interviews in Lebanon were using the term *ta'sib* to describe one of the changes that they noticed with the menopause transition. *Ta'sib* refers to an impatience and nervous tension that can grow out of control. Margaret Lock added a number of symptoms to the list of Everyday Complaints in Japan, including *katakorior* (shoulder stiffness), *miminari* (ringing in the ears), *zu chō kan* (heavy feeling in the head), *sutoresu* (stress), *seiyoku fushin* (lack of sexual desire), *handan ryoli gentai* (loss of judgment), *appakukan* (feeling of oppression), and *daeki bunpitsu zōka* (increased salivation) (Lock 1993:33–34). While Lock used three terms to measure hot flashes (*kyū na nekkan, nobose,* and *hoteri*), Melby (2005) added a fourth term, *hotto furasshu,* a word used in Japan that has been borrowed from the English term "hot flash." In Australia, Dennerstein et al. (2000) added the complaints of shortness of breath on exertion, chest pain on exertion, vaginal dryness, and breast soreness-tenderness. For the checklist used in Puebla, Mexico, the sensation of "pins and needles" was translated as *hormigueo,* or "the feeling of ants crawling on the skin," and vaginal dryness was added to the list. For the checklist used in Slovenia, we did not ask about vaginal dryness after the first dozen interviews. It became clear very quickly that the question was thought highly inappropriate by respondents because it implied sexual activity (Sievert et al. 2004).

Despite concerns about missing symptoms that are culturally defined or culturally bound, using one particular checklist across all cultures enables useful comparisons. For example, the frequency of symptoms is relatively high in Puebla, Mexico, compared with other studies. Fifty percent of the entire sample reported the experience of hot flashes during the two weeks prior to interview. Using the same checklist, hot flash frequencies were 12 percent in Japan, 31 percent in Canada, 35 percent in Massachusetts (Avis et al. 1993; Lock 1998) and 32 percent in Australia (Dennerstein et al. 1993).

Induced Menopause

As a final point related to methods and the study of menopause, we should return to the definition of menopause as the permanent cessation of menstruation due to the loss of ovarian follicular activity (WHO 1981, 1996). This definition fits the process of menopause for the majority of women in the world—the cessation of menstruation through the gradual process of follicular atresia, the depletion of oocytes (undeveloped eggs), and the eventual inability to produce the levels of ovarian hormones needed to maintain menstrual cyclicity. However, the cessation of menstruation can also occur through the loss of the uterus, through the loss of ovarian oocytes through oophorectomy (the removal of the ovaries), or through radio- or chemotherapy. Although menopause experienced because of biomedical intervention is not consistent with the WHO definition of menopause, studies of symptoms at midlife have generally included women who experienced menopause by both natural and medical means, particularly by hysterectomy and/or oophorectomy.

In population-level studies of age at menopause and symptoms associated with menopause, women who have undergone menopause by hysterectomy ("surgical menopause") are generally treated as postmenopausal even though hysterectomies without oophorectomies do not induce the hormonal changes of menopause. If menopause is defined as the end of menstruation, then a surgical menopause is menopause. Women who have had their uterus removed may still have premenopausal hormone levels; however, there is no simple way to differentiate between premenopausal and postmenopausal women (in terms of ovarian function) without a blood test for estrogen and/or FSH levels. Women who undergo menopause by hysterectomy may thus not be menopausal in a manner consistent with the WHO definition of menopause; however, in survey research they may be either excluded or treated as having undergone menopause because they are no longer menstruating. In Kaplan-Meier analyses to compute a median age at menopause, women who have undergone a hysterectomy are included in analyses up to their age at hysterectomy (described in Chapter Four). In studies of symptoms at midlife, women who have undergone menopause by medical means are either combined with postmenopausal women or given a separate category.

There are several different types of hysterectomies, but all result in the end of menstruation. In a total hysterectomy the surgeon removes the uterus and cervix. In a partial or subtotal hysterectomy the uterus is surgically removed but the cervix is left in place. Radical hysterectomies are the most extensive because they involve removal of the upper vagina and tissues surrounding the uterus as well as the uterus and cervix. Note that none of these procedures involve the ovaries. An oophorectomy is the surgical removal of the ovary.

In the 1970s bilateral oophorectomies (removal of both ovaries) were often performed with hysterectomies in the United States (Cutler and Garcia 1984). Today this practice is rare. This change in medical norms created a cohort difference that has implications for the study of menopause: one generation of women most likely underwent bilateral oophorectomies with their hysterectomies while the next generation of women did not. This difference should be kept in mind when interviewing women of different ages in any country. As discussed earlier, cohort membership shapes health behavior, diet, economic history, educational opportunities, and particular health risks—including exposure to surgical procedures. Therefore, it makes sense for researchers interested in symptom experience at menopause to ask women who have undergone a hysterectomy, "Have you ever had one or both of your ovaries removed?" [11]

In the United States, hysterectomy is currently the second most common major surgery for women of reproductive age, following Cesarean sections (Bernstein et al. 1997; Pokras and Hufnagel 1988). Each year, approximately 600,000 hysterectomies are performed in the United States (Farquhar and Steiner 2002; Lepine et al. 1997). One interesting consequence of this high frequency of hysterectomies is that younger women often face natural menopause with no guidance. In western Massachusetts, for example, women often commented that because their mothers had gone through menopause by hysterectomy, they had no one to talk to about their symptoms or experiences. They lack what is known as anticipatory guidance—help from someone who has been there, done that, before.

Leiomyoma (fibroids) are the most common indication for hysterectomy, along with abnormal uterine bleeding, endometriosis, uterine prolapse, and gynecological cancers (Lepine et al. 1997). Leiomyoma are benign tumors of the smooth muscle, in this case the smooth muscle of the uterus. Not all uterine fibroids cause symptoms, but for some women they can cause heavy menstrual bleeding that lasts for days or weeks, pelvic pressure, and pain. Fibroids can be treated with hormones (such as progesterone), but sometimes they are removed if they cause severe discomfort or extremely heavy uterine bleeding. Fibroids are sometimes removed by myomectomy (when only the tumor is removed from the uterine wall) or by hysterectomy (when the entire uterus is removed). For reasons that are not yet understood, uterine fibroids are more common in African American women than in white women (Marshall et al. 1997), and African American women having hysterectomies have larger and more numerous uterine fibroids than do white women (Kjerulff et al. 1996).

Words like leiomyoma, endometriosis, and uterine prolapse may be very familiar to the physician making the diagnosis, but the woman herself may not understand why she is undergoing the surgery. Davis (1983) found that six of her informants in Newfoundland had undergone a hysterectomy, but none knew why or whether her ovaries had also been removed. Among the reasons they gave for the hysterectomy were (1) weak insides, (2) flooding or heavy bleeding, and (3) tuberculosis or cancer of the womb.

In Puebla, Mexico, 167 women who underwent hysterectomies answered the open-ended question "Why did you have a hysterectomy?" As table 3.6 shows, the primary reason given was *mioma, fibroma,* or benign tumor, probably all references to fibroid tumors. Twenty-six women used the word *quistes* (cysts) that, though not clinically correct, probably also referred to fibroid tumors.[12] Reasons that may sound surprising to researchers in the United States included infection, miscarriage, uterine perforation (probably during childbirth), and birth control. In Asunción, Paraguay, reasons included a problem with an IUD, childbirth, and "midwife." As in Mexico and the United States, the principal reason given for a hysterectomy in Asunción was fibroid tumor.

TABLE 3.6

Reasons Given for Hysterectomies in Puebla, Mexico (*n* = 167), and Asunción, Paraguay (*n* = 62) (in Percent)

Reason	Puebla	Asunción
Mioma, fibroma, or benign tumor (fibroid tumor)	35	61
Quistes (cysts; in Paraguay also *nódulos* or *pólipos*)	16	18
Heavy bleeding	13	8
Infection	5	
Cancer	5	
Miscarriage, ectopic pregnancy, stillbirth, delivery, and uterine perforation	4	3
Uterine prolapse	4	3
Birth control	2	2
Others (including endometriosis, hyperplasia, positive pap smear, ulcer, pain, *problemas,* and don't know)	16	5

Note: These reasons were volunteered in response to an open-ended question.

Hysterectomy rates vary among countries (McPherson et al. 1982), within countries (Bernstein et al. 1992; Hall and Cohen 1994; Kjerulff, Langenberg, and Guzinski 1993; Pokras and Hufnagel 1988; Santow and Bracher 1992), and within states (Bickell et al. 1994; Hass et al. 1993; New York State 1988). Table 3.7

TABLE 3.7

Hysterectomy Rates Reported in Studies of Age at Menopause

Study Population/Site	Ages of Women in Study	Rate of Hysterectomy	Source
Australia, Brisbane	45–54	31	O'Connor et al. (1995)
Italy 1983–1992	55–74	14	Parazzini, Negri, and La Vecchia (1992)
Mexico, Puebla	28–70	23	Sievert and Hautaniemi (2003)
The Netherlands, Ede	42–62	6	Jaszmann, van Lith, and Zaat (1969)
	40–60	21	Brand and Lehert (1978)
Norway		10	Holte (1991)
Paraguay, Asunción	36–71	14	Unpublished
Portugal	38–91	12	Guedes Pinto da Cunha (1984)
UK		12	M. S. Hunter (1990)
		20	Coulter, McPherson, and Vessey (1988)
U.S., national, 1960–1962	18–79	13.2	MacMahon and Worcester (1966)
U.S., Minnesota, 1935–1980s	44–56	19	Whelan et al. (1990)
U.S., Multisite, 1973–1980	22–62	31	Stanford et al. (1987)
U.S., Mass., 1981–1986	45–55	28	McKinlay, Brambilla, and Posner (1992)
U.S., Blackfeet, 1995–1996	50–69	43	Johnston (2001)
U.S., Hawaii	mean 46.2 ± 7.4	66	Brown et al. (2001)

illustrates differences in rates of hysterectomies that have been encountered in studies of menopause in different countries and at different points in time. Note the differences in rates of hysterectomy among studies carried out in the same country, that is, United States and the Netherlands.

In the United States, some studies have indicated a higher rate of hysterectomy among nonwhite women compared with white women (Carlisle et al. 1995; Chandra 1998; Meilahn et al. 1989; Mort, Weissman, and Epstein 1994); Other investigators have demonstrated no racial or ethnic differences in hysterectomy rates (Lepine et al. 1997). There is some disagreement over whether Hispanic women have lower (Chandra 1998) or higher (Carlisle et al. 1995) rates of hysterectomy compared with non-Hispanic women. An analysis of the Hispanic Health and Nutrition Examination Survey (HHANES), 1982–1984, showed that Mexican American women had higher rates of hysterectomy than did either Puerto Rican or Cuban American women (Stroup-Benham and Trevino 1991).

From a biocultural perspective, hysterectomies are not performed solely for reasons having to do with disease states. If this were so, the range in rates of hysterectomy would not differ so dramatically across space and time. Like age at menopause, the occurrence of a hysterectomy can also be studied as a risk (Shinberg 1998), which requires a lifespan approach. For example, factors related to a higher risk of hysterectomy in the United States and Australia include lower education, occupational status, and income levels (Brett, Marsh, and Madans 1997; Kjerulff, Langenberg, and Guzinski 1993; Leidy 1999b; Marks and Shinberg 1997; Meilahn et al. 1989; Shinberg 1998); having given birth and having had three or more children (Hautaniemi and Sievert 2003; Santow and Bracher 1992); having an early age at first birth (Shinberg 1998); and use of IUD and history of miscarriage (Brett, Marsh, and Madans 1997; Geller, Burns, and Brailer 1996). According to Santow (1995), college-educated women in Australia were less often given the choice of a hysterectomy as a medical treatment and, when it was offered, better-educated women were less likely to act on the recommendation. In contrast, risk of hysterectomy does not vary by educational attainment in Finland (Luoto, Kaprio, and Uutela 1994).

In contrast to findings from the United States and Australia, Mexican American women and women in Mexico with *higher* levels of education and higher socioeconomic status are at an increased risk of hysterectomy. Among Mexican American women sampled by the Hispanic Health and Nutrition Examination Survey, 1982–1984, women who had finished sixth grade were over one and one-half times more likely to have had a hysterectomy than were women who had not finished sixth grade (Hautaniemi and Sievert 2003). Relatedly, perhaps, we also found that Mexican American women who preferred to speak English had over twice the risk of hysterectomy compared with Mexican American women who preferred to speak Spanish.

Similarly, in Puebla, Mexico, women of higher levels of education were more likely to undergo a hysterectomy (Sievert and Hautaniemi 2003). One factor explaining country-specific differences in risk factors associated with hysterectomy may be the generally low levels of education reported by Mexican American women in the HHANES sample and by women in Puebla. In Puebla, women went to school for an average of eight years. It may also be that women with more education consult with different medical practitioners. In Mexico, the health care system is divided among public health services, social security services (for example, for government employees), and private health services. Few people can afford private health services, but it may be that women with higher levels of education are at an economic level that allows them to use private health care and, relatedly, are more likely to be prescribed a hysterectomy. It would be of interest to see if hysterectomy rates vary in relation to type of health services utilized in Puebla.

A number of studies have found that tubal ligation is a risk factor for hysterectomies (Althaus 1994; Goldhaber et al. 1993; Hillis et al. 1998; Mall, Shirk, and Van Voorhis 2002). For example, Stergachis et al. (1990) studied 7,414 women aged twenty to forty-nine years who had undergone a tubal sterilization at a health maintenance organization from 1968 to 1983. Women sterilized while twenty to twenty-nine years old were 3.4 times more likely to undergo a hysterectomy later on compared with a population-based cohort of nonsterilized women. It may be that tubal ligation increases the risk for hysterectomy because of damage to tissue surrounding the fallopian tubes during the sterilization surgery. This damage may disrupt blood flow to the ovaries and may decrease hormonal communication between the ovaries and the uterus.

Alternatively, it may be that women who are willing to undergo surgery for contraception are more willing to undergo surgery for heavy bleeding (the leading cause of hysterectomy in the United States). From Australia, Santow (1994) pointed out that many of the same factors that predict sterilization also predict a hysterectomy, such as side effects from IUD use, Cesarean sections, and multiple miscarriages. In other words, "sterilization may be a response to a previously checkered reproductive career, and such a career is also conducive to hysterectomy" (Santow 1994:661). In a small study carried out in Canberra, Australia, Santow (1995) noted that it was common medical practice to recommend a tubal ligation after a Cesarean delivery. The effect of tubal sterilization on risk of hysterectomy disappeared after Cesareans were added to the statistical model.

Finally, it may be that a hysterectomy does not signify the end of fertility for women who have already ended their fertility through a sterilization procedure. Relatedly, a physician may no longer feel the need to preserve a woman's uterus if her reproductive function has already been terminated through sterilization (Rulin et al. 1993; Stergachis et al. 1990).

From a lifespan perspective, all of the risk factors for hysterectomy mentioned above occur relatively early in the lifespan (for example, having given birth, educational attainment, use of IUD) or are determined by choices and opportunities that occur at a relatively early point along the social (for example, occupational status) or reproductive trajectories (for example, tubal ligation). Of methodological concern, all of these factors are interrelated. Among women in Wisconsin, Shinberg (1998) found that lower education and early childbearing were both associated with a higher risk of hysterectomy. When both factors were included in the model predicting risk of hysterectomy, however, level of education was no longer a significant factor. According to Shinberg, "this suggests a framework for the pathways from education to surgery" (1393). A woman's level of education may thus be a risk factor for hysterectomy only because early childbearing is related both to low levels of educational attainment and to an increased risk of hysterectomy.

Level of education, access to health care, and age at childbirth are relatively easy to measure. More difficult to measure is the value of a woman's uterus. As Lynn Payer (1988) argued in her comparison of hysterectomy rates between the United States and France, some cultures value the uterus (France) and others do not (the United States). While working in France, a routine gynecologic checkup revealed a grapefruit-sized fibroid tumor in her uterus. It was removed by myomectomy, but recurred after she moved back to the United States. Payer (1988) described the following dissonance:

> In France, where great value is put on the woman's ability to bear children, hysterectomy was not even suggested as an option. Instead, the French surgeon told me I *must* have myomectomy, a major operation in which the fibroid tumor is removed while the ability to have children is preserved. I was told that six such operations could be performed without even necessitating a cesarean section were I to become pregnant. In the United States, I was put under a great deal of pressure for hysterectomy and told that a second myomectomy would be impossible. (22, emphasis in original)

Since the publication of Payer's *Medicine and Culture*, the uterus has gained more respect in the United States. It used to be thought that an aging uterus made pregnancy unlikely or impossible beyond the age of fifty (Gosden 1985; Maroulis 1991), but this view has since been challenged by successful postmenopausal pregnancies using donor eggs (Antinori et al. 1993; Sauer, Paulson, and Lobo 1992). Given appropriate hormonal assistance (Meldrum 1993), the uterus is capable of supporting a pregnancy well beyond the ticking of the ovarian "biological clock" (Levran et al. 1991; Navot et al. 1991). Perhaps it is not a coincidence that now, at the same point in time that postmenopausal pregnancy has become a reality, techniques that treat uterine fibroids without requiring the removal of the uterus (such as hormones, myomectomy, uterine artery embolization)[13] are becoming more and more common.

Women may regret having undergone menopause by hysterectomy. In Puebla, Mexico, as well as in western Massachusetts and Slovenia, I spoke with women who were bitter about having undergone what they later came to view as an unnecessary operation. Some women complained of losing interest in sex, or suffering pain during intercourse, due to the effects of a hysterectomy. Other women complained of a deeper hurt, of being treated as unnecessary by the medical establishment and by men in general. Explained one forty-eight-year-old single mother in Puebla, "When he took out my uterus, the doctor told me 'Sirve para la vida, pero después no sirve para nada' (It gives life but afterward does nothing). It is with this idea that men devalue women. They say 'No sirve para nada' (We serve no function)."

Many scholars and women's health activists have worked to reduce unnecessary hysterectomies (Fisher 1986; Payer 1987); however, unnecessary hysterectomies continue to be performed. At the same time, it is important to note that many women speak of their hysterectomy as something that "gave their life back" to them. When women give reasons for a hysterectomy, the terms *heavy bleeding* or *sangre abundante* (abundant blood) do not refer to a bad day during a regular period. These terms refer to bleeding so profuse that a woman cannot leave the house, cannot stand up after she has been seated for a fifty-minute meeting at work, cannot go to a family function for fear of bleeding through her pants or skirt. The general discomfort is magnified by the perception that menstrual blood is polluting or dirty (Delaney, Lupton, and Toth 1988).

Whatever the reason for a hysterectomy, it marks the end of menstruation and hence can be understood to be a form of menopause. As detailed in Chapter One, women in upstate New York who underwent a hysterectomy were more likely to say that menopause came too early in their life. When women undergo bilateral oophorectomy along with their hysterectomy, some almost immediately experience difficulties with hot flashes. When women do not undergo bilateral oophorectomy with their hysterectomy, they may be surprised by hot flashes later on in life when their follicle stores are naturally exhausted. One of the most common questions I hear from study participants who have undergone a hysterectomy is, "Am I going through menopause now [that is, years after the hysterectomy]?" If menopause is defined in terms of hormones, the answer may be yes. If, however, menopause is defined as the cessation of menses, then she has already undergone menopause—surgical menopause.

CHAPTER FOUR

Age at Menopause

By paying attention to the full range of human experience across populations, it is possible to ask broader questions. For example, what aspects of menopausal biology are universal—in the sense that there is little or no variation within or between populations? One common feature appears to be an upper age limit on the ability to menstruate. To my knowledge, women do not menstruate beyond the age of sixty-two without the use of cyclic HT. I have met only one woman—in upstate New York—who was still menstruating at sixty-two. Stanford et al. (1987) also cite one woman still menstruating at sixty-two. Sixty was the latest age at menopause observed in Finland (Luoto, Kaprio, and Uutela 1994) and Australia (Do et al. 1998). In Puebla, Mexico, the latest recalled age at menopause was fifty-six (table 4.1). In Asunción, Paraguay, the latest recalled age at menopause was also fifty-six, although the oldest woman who said she was still menstruating was sixty years of age.

Another broad question about age at menopause is, What cultural attributes have the same effect on biology, no matter the population? As this chapter will detail, never having been pregnant and smoking are two variables consistently associated with an earlier age at menopause (Cramer and Xu 1996; Do et al. 1998; Elias et al. 2003; Luoto, Kaprio, and Uutela 1994; Parazzini, Negri, and La Vecchia et al. 1992; Sievert and Hautaniemi 2003), and married women, cross-culturally, have a later age at menopause compared with single women (Jaszmann, van Lith, and Zaat 1969; McKinlay, Jefferys, and Thompson 1972; Neri et al. 1982; Sievert, Waddle, and Canali 2001; Stanford et al. 1987). Because the traits in question exert their effects on age at menopause at some point (age twenty? age thirty-four? age forty?) prior to the cessation of menstruation, associations between these variables and age at menopause are best understood from a lifespan approach.[1]

The average age at menopause within a population is determined by (1) the number of oocytes that women, in general, are born with, (2) the average rate at

TABLE 4.1

**Ranges in Age of Menstruating Women at
Interview and Ranges in Age at Menopause**

Country (site)	Range in Age at Interview among Menstruating Women	Range in Recalled Age at Natural Menopause	Mean Recalled Age at Natural Menopause
Asunción, Paraguay	36.5–60.3 ($n = 268$)	36–56 ($n = 132$)	47.9 (s.d. 3.7)
Massachusetts, USA	39.4–57.8 ($n = 167$)	28.5–57.1 ($n = 54$)	48.9 (s.d. 5.0)
Puebla, Mexico	28.2–56.9 ($n = 303$)	28–56 ($n = 268$)	46.7 (s.d. 4.8)
Selška Valley, Slovenia	32.7–54.2 ($n = 19$)	42–54 ($n = 32$)	50.3 (s.d. 2.9)

Source: Sievert and Hautaniemi (2003); Sievert et al. (2004); unpublished data.

which those oocytes and their follicles are lost through the process of atresia, and (3) the threshold number of ovarian follicles needed to maintain menstrual cyclicity within that population. Stated this way, the level of analysis shifts from an individual and her two ovaries to an entire population of women. This framework helps us understand interpopulation variation—why age at menopause is earlier among the Maya in Yucatán, Mexico, for example, than among urban women of Madrid, Spain (table 4.2).

To explain differences in average ages at menopause between populations, one might investigate variation in numbers of follicles at birth. A reasonable hypothesis would be that women born to poorly nourished mothers are born with fewer oocytes in their ovaries. This possibility could explain a population-level early age at menopause if many women of childbearing age were malnourished at the time of their daughter's development in utero. This question is currently a research area of great interest. Another reasonable hypothesis would be that women born to mothers who smoke are born with fewer oocytes because of the toxic effects of polycyclic aromatic hydrocarbons (in cigarette smoke) on oocytes (Baron, La Vecchia, and Levi 1990). This hypothesis, however, does not seem to hold up. For example, urban Spanish women with a later age at menopause are more likely to smoke than are rural Mexican women with an earlier age at menopause.

Population differences in average ages at menopause might instead be explained by variation in rates of follicular atresia. Rates of follicular atresia could

TABLE 4.2

Mean and Median Ages at Menopause

Country (site)	Mean Age at Menopause	Median Age at Menopause	N	Age at Interview	Surgical Menopause	Reference
Australian Twin Registry, 1980–1996		51 Kaplan-Meier	5,593	17–88	Censored	Do et al. (1998)
Finland, population register, 1989		51.0 Life table	1,505	45–64	Censored	Luoto, Kaprio, and Uutela (1994)
Italy, Milan, 1983–1989	49.4 Recall		863	55–74	Excluded	Parazzini, Negri, and La Vecchia (1992)
Mexico, rural Maya	42.0 Recall		71	33–57	—	Beyene (1986)
Mexico, Mayan villages	44.0 Recall		202	35–59	—	Canto-de-Cetina, Canto-Cetina, and Polanco-Reyes (1998)
Mexico, Progresso, 1989–1990	44.3 Recall		81	>31	Excluded	Dickinson et al. (1992)
Mexico, Mayan village/city	44.4 Recall		232	—	—	Beyene and Martin (2001)
Mexico, rural Tuxpan	46.0 Recall		330	34–56	Excluded	Aréchiga et al. (2000)

(continued)

Location and period			N	Age range		Reference
Mexico City, 1991–1992	45.0 Recall		313	26–83	Included	Parra-Cabrera et al. (1996)
Mexico City, 1990–1993	46.5 Recall		472	—	Excluded	Garrido-Latorre et al. (1996)
Mexico, Léon, Guanajuato		48.2 Probit	1,558	19–90	Excluded	Garcia Vela, Nava, and Malacara (1987)
Mexico, Léon, Guanajuato		48.5 Probit	490	35–55	Excluded	Velasco et al. (1990)
Mexico, Puebla, 1999–2000		49.6 Probit	755	28–70	Excluded	Sievert and Hautaniemi (2003)
Netherlands, Utrecht, 1975–1984	50.2 Prospective		4,686	58.2–73.9	Excluded	van Noord et al. (1997)
Portugal, urban Coimbra		47.0	137	40–60	—	Guedes Pinto da Cunha (1984)
rural Ançã		48.5 Status quo	83	40–60	—	
Puerto Rico		51.4 Probit	219	30–59	Excluded	Ortiz et al. (2003)
Spain, Basque		49.3 Probit	321	19–60	Excluded	Rebato (1988)
Spain, Madrid	50.0 Recall		300	51–75	Excluded	Prado and Canto (1999)
Spain, Madrid		51.7 Logit	300	45–55	Excluded	Reynolds and Obermeyer (2005)

TABLE 4.2
Mean and Median Ages at Menopause (continued)

Country (site)	Mean Age at Menopause	Median Age at Menopause	N	Age at Interview	Surgical Menopause	Reference
Spain, Alcobendas		51.7 Probit	927	45–61	Excluded	Bernis (2001); Varea et al. (2000)
USA, Blackfeet, Montana, 1995–1996		51.2 Status quo	120	30–93	Excluded	Johnston (2001)
USA, multicenter, 1973–1980		51.1 Life table	3,497	22–62	Censored	Stanford et al. (1987)
USA, Mass., 1982–1983		50.7 Hazard	2,014	46.5–56.5	Censored	Brambilla and McKinlay (1989)
USA, Mass., 2000		52.6 Probit	293	45–55	Excluded	Reynolds and Obermeyer (2005)
USA, Tremin Trust	50.5 (menopause limited to 44–56 years) prospective		561		Censored	Whelan et al. (1990)
Venezuela	48.9 Recall		167	29–78	Excluded	Reyes et al. 2005

Note: Dash indicates that information on how hysterectomies were handled in the study's analysis was not provided.

be influenced by marital practices through the effect of pheromones (Sievert, Waddle, and Canali 2001), discussed later in this chapter, or by odd health-related "opportunities." For example, my mother's generation grew up playing with X-ray machines in shoe stores. Children could put their feet into a machine and see their own toe bones. The machine, a wonderful marketing tool, exposed a generation of women to radiation that could have accelerated the rate of follicular atresia and resulted in an earlier age at menopause.[2]

Variation in average ages at menopause between populations might also be due to differences in the threshold number of oocytes needed to maintain menstrual cyclicity. This threshold could vary among populations that demonstrate lower or higher hormone levels across the lifespan. Peter Ellison has suggested that women who grow up under difficult circumstances, such as undernourishment, do not achieve the same high levels of estrogen during the reproductive years as do women who grow up under more favorable conditions. He explains that "the entire trajectory of lifetime ovarian function may be adjusted upward or downward in response to some characteristic feature of the environment in which a population finds itself" (Ellison 1999:194).

We will never fully understand the influence of cultural factors on biological variation until all investigators in all countries agree to measure age at menopause in the same way. Because of different educational and training opportunities across academic disciplines as well as across nations, because of differential access to statistical computer programs between first, second, and third worlds, and because of different levels of emphasis on age at menopause as a variable useful for cross-cultural comparisons, methodological inconsistencies still explain much of the cross-cultural difference in age at menopause. This chapter discusses how best to compute the average age at menopause, and examines variation in intra- and interpopulation age at menopause.

The Genetics of Menopause

Age at menopause appears to be highly heritable, that is, age at menopause is determined in large part by our genetic inheritance, although it is also influenced by the environment. Snieder, MacGregor, and Spector (1998) examined age at menopause among British monozygotic (identical) twins and dizygotic (fraternal) twins. They found that the correlation for menopausal age was greater (0.58) for monozygotic twins than for dizygotic twins (0.39). Because monozygotic twins share identical genotypes (genetic coding) and dizygotic twins, like all siblings, share just 50 percent of their genetic coding, the higher degree of correlation between the identical twins indicates that age at menopause is determined, in part, by genetics. But how much of the variation can be explained by our genes?

According to Snieder and colleagues (1998), 63 percent of the variation in age at menopause can be explained by genetic inheritance. That means that just 37 percent of the variation in age at menopause is explained by the environment (such as reproductive history and smoking habits). De Bruin et al. (2001) examined singleton sisters, dizygotic twins, and monozygotic twins to arrive at similarly high estimates of heritability for age at menopause (68 to 85 percent). Lower estimates of heritability for age at menopause (31 to 53 percent) were computed in a study of Australian twins (Treloar et al. 1998).

Jocelyn Peccei (1999) used data drawn from the Tremin Research Program on Women's Health to study twenty-one mother–daughter pairs followed prospectively until both experienced a natural menopause and ninety-six mother–daughter pairs in which all of the mothers experienced natural menopause but the daughters were still menstruating. The mother–daughter pairs demonstrated that between 40 percent and 50 percent of the variation in age at menopause could be explained by genetic inheritance.

In a study of age at menopause in Scotland and England, forty-five- to forty-nine-year-old women were asked to recall their mother's age at menopause. Those study participants who were postmenopausal were significantly more likely to recall an earlier early age at menopause for their mothers compared with mothers of study participants who were still menstruating, suggesting an intergenerational association in age at menopause (Torgerson et al. 1994). Finally, Cramer, Xu, and Harlow (1995) found that women with a family history of early menopause (before age forty-six) had three times the risk for experiencing an early menopause.

Premature Ovarian Failure

The influence of genes on age at menopause is most apparent in studies of premature ovarian failure. Premature ovarian failure is generally defined as menopause prior to the age of forty (Rebar 2000). Sometimes the cause of this very early menopause is wholly genetic, with no apparent role for the environment. For example, early age at menopause has been associated with a complete or partial deletion of the X chromosome (Fitch et al. 1982; Krauss et al. 1987). Women born with Turner's syndrome have only one X chromosome.[3] In a recent study, ovaries sampled from aborted fetuses with Turner's syndrome showed that although oogonia were found in some ovaries, the follicles did not develop through the primordial, preantral, or antral stages. The lack of a second X chromosome was thus seen to affect ovarian function (and hormonal production) as early as the fetal stage of development (Reynaud et al. 2004).

A number of case studies have shown that premature ovarian failure is a Mendelian trait (Coulam, Stringfellow, and Hoefnagel 1983; Mattison et al. 1984), meaning that the trait (early menopause) can be traced through families

(Mattison et al. 1984: 1344). Mattison and colleagues concluded that the gene for premature ovarian failure is either autosomal or (less likely) X-linked dominant (that is, if you inherit it, the trait is expressed).

The etiology or cause of premature ovarian failure can also be due to galactosemia (Kaufman et al. 1981). Normally when a person drinks milk, the body breaks the lactose sugar down into galactose and glucose. The word "galactosemia" means too much galactose in the blood, which occurs when a person either lacks the enzyme or has too little of the enzyme (known as GALT) needed to convert galactose into glucose. This accumulation of galactose is poisonous to the ovaries. The etiology of galactosemia is genetic; there is also, however, an environmental component, because the effects of galactosemia are worsened by drinking milk (Cramer et al. 1989).

About 20 percent of the time, the etiology of premature ovarian failure involves immune abnormalities (LaBarbera et al. 1988; Rebar and Connolly 1990). More specifically, one cause of premature ovarian failure appears to be antiovarian antibodies (Alper and Garner 1985; Chernyshov et al. 2001; Damewood et al. 1986; Luborsky et al. 1999; Rabinowe et al. 1989). In this instance the woman makes antibodies that attack her own ovaries.

Considering the medical disorder of premature ovarian failure is helpful in three ways. First, it allows us to consider an interesting idea proposed by Jocelyn Peccei (1995). She suggested that premature ovarian failure was potentially the way in which ovarian function became separated from the other body systems. Ovarian function ceases after fifty or sixty years, but the heart continues to pump, the lungs continue to provide oxygen to the blood, and so on. Human females have a long postreproductive life because reproductive and somatic aging became decoupled during the course of evolution.

Premature ovarian failure, now considered to be pathological, could have provided phenotypic variation on which natural selection could act. For example, Peccei (1995) proposed that if women with earlier menopause—due to a genetic mutation—had greater evolutionary success in terms of their own fertility and/or the fertility of their offspring, then it may be that premature ovarian failure initiated the "dynamic process" of the evolution of menopause (Peccei 1995:84). Once reproductive and somatic aging were decoupled, the age of onset of menopause could have gradually increased to keep pace with the dependence of hominid offspring as well as increasing lifespans (84).

A second reason premature ovarian failure is of interest is that some of the variables associated with premature ovarian failure are also associated with the timing of "normal" menopause (for example, galactosemia; Cramer et al. 1989). Third, in order to avoid the inclusion of women with pathogenic menopause, many investigators restrict studies of age at menopause to samples drawn from women who experienced menopause no earlier than age forty (Rebar 2000); in some cases an even older age limit is set.

Defining a Normal Menopause

Chapter Two discussed how the biocultural perspective can be used to evaluate the arbitrary cutoffs between normal and abnormal. Even a cursory review of the menopause literature shows that investigators are far from agreement on the cutoff along the continuum between premature ovarian failure and a "normal" age at menopause. For example, Garcia Vela, Nava, and Malacara (1987) surveyed 1,558 women aged nineteen to ninety in León, Guanajauto, Mexico, to determine the median age at menopause. They considered premature ovarian failure to occur before the age of thirty-five, and therefore included women aged thirty-five to fifty-nine in their analyses. In contrast, when Whelan et al. (1990) used Alan Treloar's prospective U.S. data to study age at menopause in relation to reproductive events, they restricted analyses to women with menopause between the ages of forty-four and fifty-six "because some women might have pathologic conditions resulting in very early or very late menopause" (626). At the opposite extreme, Elias et al. (2003) excluded women who reported "an unlikely age at menopause" of before twenty-four or after sixty-two.

In a study of 8,000 women aged forty-five to fifty-four in the United States, Cramer and Xu (1996) found that 2,783 had experienced menopause and that the probability of menopause before age forty was about 1 percent. The probability of menopause before age forty-five was about 5 percent. Why should we be concerned about the cutoffs? Because distribution in age at menopause varies between populations. In addition to average ages at menopause, the distribution in ages at menopause is also an aspect of human variation.[4]

If arbitrary cutoffs are set too high, then we miss an understanding of human variation by labeling and excluding more women as having premature ovarian failure in some countries compared with others. For example, the Minnesota sample used by Whelan et al. (1990) and the Boston sample used by Cramer and Xu (1996) are both drawn from relatively privileged, developed-world populations. Applying a late cutoff for age at menopause, say, forty-four or forty-five, excludes few women from the analyses. However, if the median recalled age of menopause in Chile is forty-seven, then half of the women have stopped menstruating by forty-seven and a cutoff of forty-four or forty-five would exclude a large part of the sample. In response, Gonzales and Villena (1997) have argued that the definition of menopause (as separate from premature ovarian failure) should be corrected for populations living in developing nations.

In Puebla, Mexico, 7.5 percent of naturally postmenopausal women reported menopause prior to age forty and 29 percent reported menopause prior to age forty-five (figure 2.5). In Asunción, 6 percent of naturally postmenopausal women reported menopause prior to age forty and 12 percent reported menopause prior to age forty-five (figure 4.1). What is a "normal" menopause in these populations?

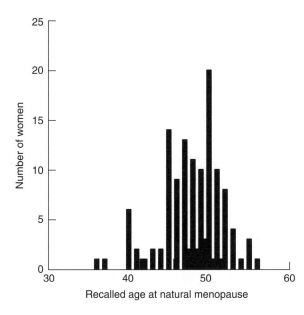

FIGURE 4.1 Recalled ages at natural menopause among women in Asunción, Paraguay.

To fully understand menopause as an aspect of human variation, we should include all ages at menopause beginning at age thirty-five.

Defining Menopause in Studies of Age at Menopause

Determining the average age at final menstruation for a population is much more difficult than determining the average age at first menstruation, for several reasons. In noncontracepting populations with prolonged lactation (breast-feeding), women may be amenorrheic for a year or longer and then experience a menstrual period—or never menstruate again (Hall 2004). Also, there are no culturally prescribed rituals associated with the last menstrual period to help identify the event. In addition, for many women across the world, menstrual cycles become increasingly irregular with age. Mitchell, Woods, and Mariella (2000) used prospective data from the Seattle Midlife Women's Health Study, described in Chapter Three, to demonstrate that midlife women reported menstrual changes—generally shorter cycles and lighter or heavier flow—as early as age thirty or as late as age fifty-four, although 41 percent reported the initial change to have occurred between ages forty and forty-four.

As women's periods become increasingly irregular, sometimes skipping three or more months between cycles, it becomes harder for them to remember when the last menstrual period occurred. This problem of remembering when menses stopped needs to be kept in mind when considering recalled ages at menopause. A dramatic exception to this blurring of memory occurs when a woman associates her last menstrual period with a traumatic event, such as the death of a loved one. Dona Lee Davis (1983) recounts how, in a Newfoundland fishing village, fright or shock was thought to result instantly in menopause. To illustrate this point, Davis quoted the following two examples: "When my daughter hemorrhaged with her first pregnancy, I took such a fright it was the last time I ever bled myself"; and "when they came and told me my husband was dead, I fainted dead away and flooded over everything. That's the last I ever saw of it [menstrual blood]" (140–141).

Among the Aché in Paraguay, one woman similarly recounted that her last menstrual period at age thirty-eight coincided with the death of her son (A. Magdalena Hurtado, personal communication). Although quite dramatic for the woman experiencing the change, the phenomenon of sudden menopause is seldom mentioned in the medical literature. Speaking about traumas that occur after menopause, Gillian Ford suggests that "many women function well after menopause until they experience a shock or trauma such as a car accident or the death of a close family member, which may bring on adrenal exhaustion" (G. Ford 1993:35). Her idea is that the adrenal glands function as backup sex organs, producing androstenedione (a precursor to the production of estrone), among other hormones. Adrenals also produce stress hormones, such as cortisol. This proposed connection between the adrenal glands and difficulty at menopause is provocative, and further investigation is needed.

Some investigators, unsatisfied with the dichotomy of categorizing women as pre- versus postmenopausal have proposed stages to better describe the menopause transition. To that end, the Stages of Reproductive Aging Workshop (STRAW) was convened in Park City, Utah, in July 2001 by the National Institutes of Health, the North American Menopause Society, and the American Society for Reproductive Medicine (Utian 2001). The twenty-seven invited participants included investigators involved with studies detailed in Chapter Three, such as the Melbourne Women's Midlife Health Project (Lorraine Dennerstein), the Seattle Midlife Study (Ellen Mitchell and Nancy Woods), the Massachusetts Women's Health Study (Nancy Avis), the Tremin Research Program (Kathleen O'Connor), and the SWAN study (Gail Greendale, Sioban Harlow, Sybil Crawford, and others). The resulting stages of normal reproductive aging are shown in table 4.3 (Soules et al. 2001).

The STRAW system, however, is not to be applied in the following circumstances: cigarette smoking, extremes of body weight (BMI greater than 30 kg/m²), heavy exercise (more than 10 h/wk of aerobic exercise), chronic menstrual cycle irregularity, prior hysterectomy, abnormal uterine anatomy (for example, fibroids), or abnormal ovarian anatomy (for example, endometrioma) (Soules et al. 2001). These circumstances are not uncommon. In 1998, 22 percent of the women in the United States smoked cigarettes (CDC 2001). This percentage is much higher in some countries, such as Lebanon (Obermeyer, Ghorayeb, and Reynolds 1999). At the present time, more than 30 percent of the U.S. population has a BMI greater

TABLE 4.3

Stages/Nomenclature of Normal Reproductive Aging in Women

Stage	Duration	Menstrual Cycles	Endocrine Characteristics
Reproductive			
Early	Variable	Variable to regular	Normal FSH
Peak	Variable	Regular	Normal FSH
Late	Variable	Regular	Elevated FSH
Menopausal transition			
Early (perimenopause)	Variable	Variable cycle length (more than seven days' difference in length of menstrual cycles)	Elevated FSH
Late[a] (perimenopause)	Variable	Two or more skipped cycles (no bleeding for more than sixty days)	Elevated FSH
Postmenopause			
Early[a] (perimenopause first year)	Five years following last menstruation	None	Elevated FSH
Late	Until demise	None	Elevated FSH

[a] Stages most likely to be characterized by hot flashes.

than 30 kg/m^2, and estimates are that by the year 2008, 300 million people world-wide will have BMIs in excess of 30 kg/m^2 (Hill et al. 2003). Women are more likely than men to be obese (Brown and Konnor 1987). Heavy labor is a central part of women's lives in much of the developing world, for example in Nepal (Panter-Brick and Pollard 1999). Menstruation is not a monthly occurrence in populations that have high parity rates (number of children) and long periods of breastfeeding (Ellison 2001a; Wood 1994). In addition, 37 percent of women in the United States undergo a hysterectomy prior to the age of sixty (Farquhar and Steiner 2002; Pokras and Hufnagel 1988). In other words, the women who fit the criteria for the staging system described in table 4.3 are nonsmoking, low parity, relatively healthy women living sedentary lifestyles who still have a uterus intact. The staging system may not be as useful for investigators working in more diverse populations.

Another concern is the reliance on FSH levels (from venous blood obtained between cycle days two and five) as a stage marker. These data may be difficult to impossible to obtain for researchers in countries lacking an infrastructure that supports health-related research. STRAW participants apparently reached a consensus that "serum FSH immunoassays are readily available and relatively inexpensive" (Soules et al. 2001:404). What may seem inexpensive to Australian, Canadian, United States, and western European researchers, however, may be far out of reach for colleagues in developing countries.

Admittedly, the staging system/nomenclature is a "work in progress" (Soules et al. 2001:405) that is still fielding comments and critiques (den Tonkelaar et al. 2002; Soules et al. 2002). The exercise of creating a staging system illustrates the difficulties inherent in the study of menopause as a universal (species-level) and global phenomenon. As biological anthropologists have repeatedly demonstrated, cross-cultural comparisons of morphological and physiological variation are best achieved through simple and accessible measures. Requiring FSH levels to be part of a staging system will certainly offer more precise information, cross-culturally, than is now available regarding the details of the menopausal transition, and will improve comparability of symptom experience during the menopause transition. Cost and logistics, however, will limit the use of this staging system to well-funded, biomedically oriented researchers.

Methods for Computing an Average Age at Menopause

As table 4.2 shows, age at menopause varies widely across populations. For example, in the United States median ages at menopause fall between forty-nine and fifty-two years (Brambilla and McKinlay 1989; Stanford et al. 1987). In contrast, mean age at menopause is forty-four years in Yucatán, Mexico (Beyene and Martin 2001; Canto-de-Cetina, Canto-Cetina, and Polanco-Reyes 1998; Dickinson et al. 1992). In general, average age at menopause appears to be earlier in developing countries than in highly westernized countries. But a number of methodological reasons may explain why this appears to be so, all having to do with the comparability of information (Morabia et al. 1998; Thomas et al. 2001). First, there may be differences in the definition of menopause. Second, there may be differences in the inclusion or exclusion of women with hysterectomies. Third, there are most certainly differences in methods of analysis.

Different definitions of menopause confound cross-study comparability (Kaufert et al. 1986). Currently most investigators use the definition of menopause as the last menstrual period (LMP) followed by twelve months of amenorrhea (WHO 1996), although some studies have defined menopause as not having menstruated for three months (Stanford et al. 1987) or six months (Beyene 1986) prior to interview. While some researchers note that few women in their late forties experience the return of regular menstruation after six months of amenorrhea (Cramer and Xu 1996), ovarian follicles continue to develop in the ovaries of women well into their fifties, as noted in Chapter One. Although not common, menstruation can return after six months of amenorrhea (Holman et al. 2002; Kaufert, Gilbert, and Tate 1987). This area needs further research.

The second issue clouding comparisons of age at menopause across populations is the decision to include or exclude women with hysterectomies. For example, mean age at menopause in Mexico City was calculated to be both 46.5 years (s.d. 5.0) (Garrido-Latorre et al. 1996) and 45.0 years (s.d. 6.7) (Parra-Cabrera et al. 1996)—a difference of 1.5 years. How did this happen? The first study excluded women with hysterectomies; the second study included participants who underwent menopause by hysterectomy (48 percent of the postmenopausal women). The early mean age at hysterectomy (41.0 years) lowered the mean age at menopause. For this reason, hysterectomies are generally excluded from studies of mean and median ages at menopause (Kaufert et al. 1986) unless the analysis is a life table analysis, discussed below.

The third source of difficulty for cross-population comparisons arises from the use of different methods to compute age at menopause. The majority of studies carried out in developing countries, with few exceptions (Garcia Vela, Nava, and Malacara 1987; Sievert and Hautaniemi 2003; Velasco et al. 1990), report mean recalled age at menopause. A mean age at menopause is computed as the average age at menopause recalled by postmenopausal women. At times, mean age at menopause is computed from prospective data, where women are followed until they experience menopause. In contrast to mean ages at menopause, the majority of studies carried out in highly westernized countries compute a median age at menopause by probit analysis (Malacara 1998) or life table analysis (Do et al. 1998; Luoto, Kaprio, and Uutela 1994; Stanford et al. 1987). Median ages at menopause are found by asking all women if they are or are not menstruating, then computing the point at which 50 percent of women are menstruating and 50 percent of women are not.

Susan Hautaniemi Leonard and I applied three different methodologies to the same data set to find the average age of menopause in Puebla, Mexico. First, we found that mean recalled age at natural menopause was 46.7 years (when all ages at menopause were included). Second, we found that the median age at menopause computed by probit analysis was 49.6 years. Third, we found that the median age at menopause as computed by Kaplan-Meier survival analysis was 50.0 years (Sievert and Hautaniemi 2003). So how do we decide which number is the average age at menopause? What are the strengths and limitations of each of these methods?

Prospective Studies of Age at Menopause

As a number of investigators have noted (Cramer and Xu 1996; Luoto, Kaprio, and Uutela 1994), the ideal population for studying age at menopause is premenopausal women in their late thirties who can be followed for fifteen or twenty years as they move through the menopause transition. As detailed in the last chapter, Alan Treloar initiated the first prospective study of menopause by following a cohort of women from their college years in Minnesota in the 1930s until 1981, when he was able to publish a mean age of 49.5 years for the 763 women who reached either a natural or a surgical menopause. In this study women were followed until they stopped menstruating; their age at menopause was noted and averaged into the mean. Elizabeth Whelan and colleagues (1990) used the same data, but reported a different age at menopause for the sample because they restricted age at menopause to between forty-four and fifty-six years and they corrected for hysterectomy as an independent competing risk (for the cessation of menses). Consequently, their estimated mean age at natural menopause for 561 women drawn from the same data was older, 50.5 years.

A less ideal, but similarly longitudinal study of age at menopause was carried out by van Noord et al. (1997) and Elias et al. (2003). These researchers followed three cohorts of Dutch women born between 1911 and 1941 from an initial screening from 1975 to 1977 (when the first cohort was aged fifty to sixty-six) through as many as five follow-ups. However, even with the prospective design, 79.5 percent of the study population reported their ages at menopause retrospectively (Elias et al. 2003).

Mean Recalled Age at Menopause

To compute a mean recalled age at menopause from cross-sectional data (as in Puebla, Mexico), postmenopausal women are asked to remember when they last menstruated. Their ages at last menstruation are then averaged together. Although this is the easiest way to compute an average age at menopause, there are problems. First, mean age at menopause is underestimated for a population when the sample includes a large proportion of women under the age of fifty, because women who continue to menstruate to later ages are lost to analysis (Cramer and Xu 1996; Bernis 2001). On the other hand, samples that include a large proportion of women over the age of fifty-five risk recall error because many women will have not menstruated for many years (Bean et al. 1979; Colditz et al. 1987; Gray 1976; Hahn, Eaker, and Rolka 1997; McKinlay and McKinlay 1973). At times, error in recall is visible in data clustering at ages forty-five, fifty, or fifty-two (Cramer and Xu 1996; Garcia Vela, Nava, and Malacara 1987; Gray 1976; Luoto, Kaprio, and Uutela 1994; WHO 1996). For example, figure 2.5 shows the distribution in recalled ages at menopause among the women interviewed in Puebla ($n = 451$). Age clustering was apparent at forty, forty-five, and fifty years. Figure 4.1 shows the distribution in recalled ages at menopause among women in Asunción, Paraguay ($n = 132$). Age clustering is less apparent at ages forty and forty-five, although quite visible at age fifty.

Rodstrom et al. (2005) studied recall error among 565 women in Goteborg, Sweden, who reported their age at menopause sometime between 1968 and 1981, then again in 1992. Over half (56 percent) of the participants in 1992 recalled an

TABLE 4.4

Mean Recalled Age at Menopause in Puebla, Mexico

Recalled Age at Menopause, Puebla, Mexico *(Age at Interview 39.75–70.1)*	*Mean (s.d.)*
Natural (age at menopause 28–56)	46.7 (4.77)
Natural (limiting sample to women with an age at menopause of 40–56)	47.6 (3.81)
Natural or surgical (age at menopause 25–58)	44.8 (5.87)
Natural or surgical (limiting sample to women with an age at menopause 40–58)	46.9 (3.97)

Source: Sievert and Hautaniemi (2003).

age at menopause that fell within one year of their first report. However, women with an early menopause (under forty-five years) tended to remember a later age at menopause, and women with a late menopause (over fifty-five years) tended to remember an earlier age at menopause.

Table 4.4 shows results from our efforts to compute a mean recalled age at natural menopause in Puebla, Mexico (Sievert and Hautaniemi 2003). Mean recalled age at natural menopause for all women reporting menopause was 46.7. However, when women reporting a natural menopause prior to age forty were excluded (to avoid including women with premature ovarian failure), mean recalled age at natural menopause rose to 47.6 years, with less variance around the mean. This demonstrates the effect of different age cutoffs on mean age at menopause. As noted above, in countries where the range in "normal" ages at menopause may extend to ages earlier than forty, the truncation of data at forty (or thirty-five as in the case of Garcia Vela, Nava, and Malacara 1987) may distort the picture. As expected, when women with hysterectomies were included in the sample, the mean age at menopause was lower ($p < .01$). The estimate without age restriction was more strongly affected, because ages at hysterectomy were relatively low. Ages at hysterectomy ranged from twenty-five to fifty-eight, with a mean of 41.8 years (s.d. 6.2).

Median Age at Menopause by Probit Analysis

A better estimate of age at menopause in cross-sectional studies is the median age at natural menopause as computed by probit analysis (Bernis 2001; Finney 1962; Gray 1976). Probit analysis is a status quo technique, a type of regression analysis where menstrual status at interview is the dependent variable and age at interview is the predictor. It estimates the point at which half of the women in a population have had menopause, and half of the women have not, assuming a normal distribution in age at menopause (figure 3.2). This method avoids any reliance on women's memory, therefore there is no error due to faulty recall of age at menopause. However, the median age at menopause computed by probit analysis can reflect the age distribution of the sample (ages at interview). Studies in which the sample contains a greater proportion of young women may generate a younger age at menopause, regardless of the timing of menopause in the population.

To obtain the proper estimate of the median age at menopause, the sample must either be representative of the larger population or be weighted to standardize the sample to the age distribution of the population as a whole. In Puebla, Mexico, Susan Hautaniemi Leonard weighted the sample to the age distribution of the population of the state of Puebla (Sievert and Hautaniemi 2003). Table 4.5 shows how limiting age at menopause to forty or older (to exclude women with premature ovarian failure) slightly increased the median age at menopause from 49.6 to 50.1 years by changing the ages at interview. As with mean age at menopause, the inclusion of women with hysterectomies lowered the median age at menopause by about two years.

Median Age at Menopause by Life Table Analysis

Some investigators argue that the best estimate of a median age at menopause is that calculated by Kaplan-Meier cumulative survivorship estimates (Cramer and

---

TABLE 4.5

Median Age at Menopause by Probit Analysis in Puebla, Mexico

Probit Estimates of Age at Menopause	Age at Interview	Age at Menopause	Median Age at Menopause (Std. Error)
Natural	39.75–70.1	28–56	49.6 (.079)
Natural	44.6–70.1	Sample limited to women with an age at menopause of 40–56	50.1 (.078)
Natural or surgical	39.5–70.1	25–58	47.5 (.072)

Source: Sievert and Hautaniemi (2003).

Xu 1996). Kaplan-Meier estimation makes no assumptions about the underlying distribution of age at menopause and includes censored cases over the span of their observation. Thus even though naturally menopausal women are the response group (Luoto, Kaprio, Uutela 1994), the experience of premenopausal women is included until the date of their last menstrual period. The information from premenopausal women is valuable because they have not stopped menstruating and, using Kaplan-Meier analyses, their information is used, not excluded as in analyses of mean recalled age at natural menopause. Similarly, the experience of women who underwent menopause by hysterectomy is also included until the date of their hysterectomy (Shinberg 1998). Their years of menstruation are not completely lost from the analysis because these women are not excluded at the beginning of the analysis as they are from the computation of mean recalled age at natural menopause and median age at natural menopause by probit analysis. Premenopausal women and women who underwent a surgical menopause are censored (taken out of the analyses) at the date of their last menstrual period or at their age of hysterectomy (Stanford et al. 1987).

A type of life table analysis, Kaplan-Meier estimates the cumulative probability of not having undergone menopause up to a given age over the course of the life span, based on exposure to the possibility of menopause at each age (Lee 1980). Figure 4.2 shows the proportion of women who continue to menstruate by age.

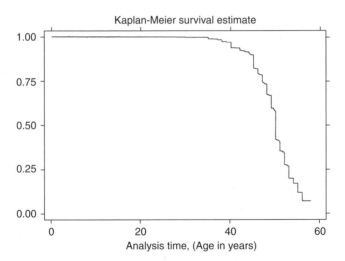

FIGURE 4.2 Kaplan-Meier life table analysis was used to compute median age at menopause in Puebla, Mexico. The line shows the decline in the number of women "surviving." In this case, surviving means still menstruating. The terminology is misleading; postmenopausal women aren't "dead." As with the probit analysis illustrated in figure 3.2, look for the halfway point along the survival estimate; that point, at 50.0 years, is the median age at menopause.

Source: Courtesy of Susan Hautaniemi Leonard.

This method is especially suitable for small populations and produces an accurate estimate of median age at menopause (Sievert and Hautaniemi 2003). A limitation of this method is that it relies on recalled ages at menopause from postmenopausal study participants. As with mean ages at menopause, this reliance on recall introduces the problems discussed above of data clustering and regression toward the mean (women with an early menopause remembering a later age at menopause, and women with a late menopause remembering an earlier age at menopause).

In Puebla, Mexico, Susan Hautaniemi Leonard used Kaplan-Meier life table analyses to obtain median ages at menopause of fifty years whether hysterectomies were censored or excluded, but with greater precision (that is, a smaller confidence interval) under censoring (table 4.6). Limiting natural menopause to begin at forty made almost no difference in the survival estimate (50.0, 95% CI 50.0–50.2). Treating both natural menopause and menopause by hysterectomy as a response group lowered the median age at menopause to forty-eight.

In summary, comparisons of age at menopause between populations are made difficult by the different methodologies used. In Puebla, Mexico, Susan Hautaniemi Leonard and I applied three different methodologies to the same data set and arrived at three different averages (46.7, 49.6, and 50.0) for age at menopause in the same population (Sievert and Hautaniemi 2003). The better estimates of age at menopause in Puebla suggest that the average age at menopause (49.6 or 50.0 years) in urban Mexico is not much earlier than average ages at menopause in the United States or Europe.

TABLE 4.6

**Median Age at Menopause in Puebla, Mexico,
by Kaplan-Meier Life Table Analysis**

| *Kaplan-Meier Cumulative Survivorship Estimates* | *Median* |
(Age at Interview 28.2–70.1*)*	*(95% CI)*
Natural, hysterectomies censored	50
(age at menopause 25–58)	(50–50)
Natural, hysterectomies excluded	50
(age at menopause 28–56)	(49–50)
Natural or surgical	48
(age at menopause 25–58)	(48–49)

Source: Sievert and Hautaniemi (2003).

Variation in Age at Menopause

As table 4.2 shows, there is a wide range of variation in age at menopause. This global overview allows us to search for some broad patterns. For example, has there been a secular trend in age at menopause? A secular trend is a gradual, unidirectional change in a characteristic over time. The word "secular" is related to the Latin word for "century" *(saeculum);* therefore a secular trend is one that takes place over one hundred years or over two or three generations.[5] For example, ages at menarche have become earlier over time (Eveleth and Tanner 1990) and height has increased over time (Bogin 1999). However, such a secular trend has seldom been convincingly demonstrated for age at menopause (Flint 1997). In a study carried out in Goteborg, Sweden, by Rodstrom et al. (2003), ages at menopause recalled by women born in 1908, 1914, 1918, 1922, and 1930 suggest an upward trend in age at menopause of 0.1 years per birth year. It is much harder to demonstrate a secular trend in age at menopause, however, if the data were collected at different times by different investigators, because of different methods of analysis used. In Finland, for example, in 1961, mean age at natural menopause was estimated to be 49.8 years, somewhat earlier than the recent median age at natural menopause of 51 years estimated by Kaplan-Meier analysis (Luoto, Kaprio, and Uutela 1994). Although it appears that the average age at menopause is now later in Finland, as the previous discussion emphasized, different methods of analysis do not give comparable results.

Peccei (1999) gives three possible explanations for the apparent lack of a secular trend in age at menopause. First, age at menopause may be under "stabilizing selection," which means that in contemporary populations there must be some cost to prolonging fertility. Second, there may be no selection on the mean age at menopause within a population. Or third, there may be an upward trend, but present data cannot show it. Thomas et al. (2001) suggest that the secular trend in age at menarche occurs because age at menarche is mainly determined by extrinsic factors such as living conditions. In contrast, they argue, age at menopause seems to be mainly influenced by intrinsic factors. This last point is somewhat controversial, as the next section demonstrates.

Factors Associated with Age at Menopause

As we have seen, age at menopause is determined by the number of eggs a woman is born with, the rate of loss of those eggs across the entire lifespan, and the threshold number of ovarian follicles required to maintain menstrual cyclicity. Mathematical models suggest that age at menopause is more sensitive to changes in rates of atresia than to differences in the initial number of oocytes (Thomford, Jelovsek, and Mattison 1987). Therefore, although there are likely factors that increase or decrease the number of eggs that develop during the fetal period, in order to understand the effects of culture-specific behaviors or stress on age at menopause, it is probably most biologically relevant to focus on factors that increase or decrease the rate of atresia (degeneration of ovarian follicles) before birth, before puberty, and before menopause (see figure 1.4).

The identification of these factors involves some leaps of biological faith, because there are no windows into ovarian physiology along the way except for those afforded by the extreme measures of autopsy (Reynaud et al. 2004) or ovarian biopsy, the less precise measure of ultrasonography (Wallace and Kelsey 2004; Flaws et al. 2001), or the actual occurrence of menopause. Therefore, to say that any one factor (for example, childhood nutrition) has an effect on oocyte numbers or rate of follicular atresia involves quite a bit of educated guesswork.

Another complication is that factors associated with age at menopause are interrelated. For example, in Puebla, education raises the age at menopause and smoking lowers it (Sievert and Hautaniemi 2003). Each variable can be examined independently with age at menopause to determine its effect, but the best way to understand the effects of all factors together is through multivariate analyses, such as Cox proportional hazards regression (Luoto, Kaprio, and Uutela 1994).[6] This statistical technique limits factors to only those characteristics that were fixed prior to or throughout exposure to the risk of menopause. In other words, we can only ask about smoking prior to menopause, marital status prior to menopause, or BMI prior to menopause, to understand the effects of these factors on age at menopause. In Puebla, we asked women if they were currently smoking, and if so, for how many years. This information was used, along with age at menopause, to identify women who were known to be smoking before menopause. These details turned out to be important, because a surprising number of women began smoking at or around the time of menopause—in part to control weight gain.

The following factors are thought to be associated with age at menopause.

Childhood Nutrition

There has been a long-standing assumption that women in poor nutritional circumstances will have an earlier age at menopause (Frisch 1978; Gray 1976; Wood 1994). Rose Frisch (1978) made this argument by comparing contemporary well-nourished Hutterite women with poorly nourished, mid-nineteenth-century Scottish women. According to Frisch, the "longer reproductive span of the modern well-nourished population reflects the secular trend to an earlier menarche and later menopause associated with better nutrition, more rapid growth in height and weight, and earlier attainment of adult size" (23). Comparisons between contemporary populations also suggest that well-nourished westernized populations enjoy a later age at menopause (table 4.2); however, as detailed above, much of the difference in age at menopause between developed and developing nations can be attributed to the different methods used to compute average age at menopause.

Turning to evidence for the effect of nutritional status on age at menopause *within* populations, Shinberg (1998) used the Wisconsin Longitudinal sample to show that having a father who was a farmer was associated with a later age at menopause. She concluded that a "farm background may be indicative of health-related lifestyle factors, including nutrition" (1393). Susan Johnston (2001) found that Blackfeet women in Montana with later ages at menarche reported earlier ages at menopause. She hypothesized that the negative association between ages at menarche and menopause would be strongest within populations that were nutritionally stressed early in life, perhaps through mechanisms that affected ovarian function. More specifically, the Blackfeet women were born to nutritionally compromised mothers and grew up during a time of episodic food shortages due to drought, bad winters, and economic crises. Tuberculosis was rampant, health care was inadequate, and most women did heavy physical labor (Johnston 2001).

Elias et al. (2003) examined age at natural menopause among women in the Netherlands who had been exposed to severe famine conditions during the last year of World War II. In January 1945, the official daily ration of food per capita for adults was below 700 kilocalories. Exposure categories (severely exposed, moderately exposed, unexposed) were constructed from memories of hunger, cold, and weight loss—hardly, little, or very much. Women were considered to be "severely exposed" if they reported "very much" exposure to at least two of the famine characteristics. "Moderately exposed" women experienced at least a "little" of two of the famine characteristics.

Elias et al. (2003) found that women who were severely exposed to famine conditions experienced natural menopause, on average, 0.37 years earlier than women who were not exposed. The effects persisted after adjusting for smoking, socioeconomic status, parity, BMI, age at menarche, and year of birth. The investigators were also able to divide participants into subgroups according to their age at the start of the famine (October 1, 1944). Exposure during early childhood had stronger effects; women who were severely exposed from ages two to six years demonstrated a decrease in age at menopause of 1.83 years compared with the unexposed group. Women who were severely exposed from seven to nine years of age demonstrated a decrease in age of menopause of 1.3 years. Exposure during adulthood resulted in a 0.14-year decline in age at menopause compared with women who were not exposed. Does this support the hypothesis that age at menopause is earlier in poorly nourished women?

Among women who reported being moderately exposed to famine conditions, mean age at natural menopause was only 0.08 years earlier than the unexposed group. Again, exposure during early childhood (two to nine years) had the strongest effect (between 0.16 and 0.22 years). However, moderate exposure to famine conditions after the age at nine had almost no effect at all (Elias et al. 2003). In other words, it appears that the exposure to hunger, cold, and weight loss had to be quite severe to have an effect.

This conclusion is consistent with the findings of Azucena Barroso Benítez (2003), who studied age at menopause in relation to the Spanish Civil War and found no significant effect of the war on age at menopause. In Britain, a National Survey of Health and Development has been following a cohort of women from their birth in 1946 through menopause and beyond (Wadsworth 1991). The researchers found no relationship between birth weight and age at menopause (Hardy and Kuh 2002b), which is consistent with other studies (Cresswell et al. 1997; Treloar et al. 2000). Instead, they demonstrated a positive relationship between childhood weight at age two and age at menopause. The authors suggested that the relationship between weight at age two and age at menopause represented a postnatal influence on ovarian function, possibly early nutrition (breastfeeding). There was no relationship between childhood weight at age seven and age at menopause (Hardy and Kuh 2002b).

In Puebla, we were unable to demonstrate an effect of childhood diet on age at menopause. Women were asked, "When you were a child of five to ten years of age, how many times per week did you eat . . . ?" Eight food items were listed, including meat, milk, and chicken. The distribution of answers was bimodal; in general, women reported an intake of zero to four times or seven times per week for each food item queried.[7] These measures of childhood nutrition did not, however, explain variation in age at menopause (Sievert and Hautaniemi 2003).

A variable that was significant in explaining age at menopause was BMI at age eighteen. In addition to food recall, women were asked to recall their weight at age eighteen. There was some clustering at 40 kg (8 percent), 45 kg (14 percent), 48 kg (8 percent), and 50 kg (10 percent); however, the answers were normally distributed. We assumed that changes in height were not substantial by the age of sixty, and therefore BMI at age eighteen was determined by recalled weight divided by height at interview squared (Bernis 1997). We found that the effect of being overweight or obese at age eighteen lowered the age at menopause (Sievert and Hautaniemi 2003).

This conclusion seems to be inconsistent with the assumption of an earlier age at menopause among poorly nourished women. Elias et al. (2003) suggest that caloric restriction may accelerate the loss of ovarian follicles through atresia, leading to an earlier menopause. However, scientists working to understand ovarian follicles have not found a mechanism for such a process. In his book *Physiology of the Graafian Follicle and Ovulation*, R.H.F. Hunter (2003) suggests only that nutrition may play a role in the regulation of insulin-like growth factor (IGF-I). If IGF-I synthesis by the granulosa cells of the ovary is disrupted, then this could impair the maturation of ovarian follicles. Elias et al. (2003) also hypothesize that caloric restriction may cause changes in neuroendocrine pathways. In this case, both severe famine and obesity might have the same effect of disrupting neuroendocrine cycles, somehow speeding up the rate of ovarian atresia and the exhaustion of ovarian follicles (Leidy 1996b).

Infectious Disease

Few studies have examined the link between infectious disease and age at menopause. Cramer et al. (1983) observed a negative correlation between ages at menarche and menopause among women who had been exposed to mumps, suggesting that the mumps virus could accelerate the rate of atresia, leading to an earlier age at menopause. No other infectious disease has been associated with age at menopause, although pelvic inflammatory disease could also be associated with age at menopause if the ovaries become involved (Daniel W. Cramer, personal communication).

Socioeconomic Status and Level of Education

Most studies of age at menopause have found that women of lower socioeconomic status experience an earlier age at menopause compared with women of higher socioeconomic status (Garrido-Latorre et al. 1996; Johnston 2001; Stanford et al. 1987). One methodological quirk, however, is that investigators define socioeconomic status in different ways. For example, in the Netherlands, Elias et al. (2003) based socioeconomic status on type of health insurance: public (lower status), civil servant's (intermediate status), or private (high status). They found that age at menopause was earliest in the lower-status group. Other investigators use current household income. Hardy and Kuh (2005) found that age at menopause was earlier among British women whose fathers were in a manual occupation during their childhood compared with women whose fathers were in nonmanual occupations. Many investigators use level of education as a measure of socioeconomic status and find that women with lower levels of education experience an earlier age at menopause (Brambilla and McKinlay 1989; Cramer and Xu 1996; Luoto, Kaprio, and Uutela 1994; Parazzini, Negri, and La Vecchia 1992; Sievert and Hautaniemi 2003).

Different explanations have been given for the relationship between education and age at menopause. In Finland, Luoto and colleagues (1994) thought that perhaps upper-class women participated in more strenuous sports activities during leisure time, producing more anovulatory cycles and thus a later age at menopause. The problem with linking age at menopause to frequency of ovulation is that only 0.1 percent of the human female's enormous supply of ovarian follicles are lost to ovulation. The rest are lost through the process of atresia. Speeding up or slowing down ovulation would have little effect on age at menopause unless the rate of atresia also changed.

Another explanation for the relationship between education and age at menopause is that women with more education are less likely to smoke, and therefore the effect of education is explained by smoking (Brambilla and McKinlay 1989; Shinberg 1998). This may be true in some populations, but the association between education and age at menopause was not confounded by smoking effects in Finland (Luoto, Kaprio, and Uutela 1994) or Italy (Parazzini, Negri, and

La Vecchia 1992), and in Mexico women of higher education are *more* likely to smoke.

Perhaps the association between age at menopause and level of education is explained by nutritional status (Stanford et al. 1987), reproductive choices, or stress (Shinberg 1998). Probably the most interesting explanation offered comes from the work of Shinberg (1998), who used the Wisconsin Longitudinal sample. She looked at mental ability (measured in terms of school grades, class rank, and intelligence scores)[8] rather than years of education and found that women with higher levels of ability had a later age at menopause.

Marital Status

Consistently, cross-culturally, never-married women report an earlier age at menopause (reviewed in Sievert, Waddle, and Canali 2001). Some researchers have suggested sexual activity as a causal connection between marital status and age at menopause (Jaszmann, van Lith, and Zoat 1969; McKinlay, Jefferys, and Thompson 1972). Others have looked to parity and use of oral contraceptives to explain the relationship (Stanford et al. 1987). Income levels may play a confounding role. The explanation that I favor is that the presence of a male in the household affects age at menopause through the influence of primer pheromones. Primer pheromones are chemicals that exert an indirect influence on the physiology of others (Weller 1998). Diane Waddle, Kris Canali, and I proposed this explanation, in part, because it is consistent with the observation that female rats housed with male rats demonstrate a longer cycling lifespan (Nass, Lapolt, and Lu 1982). Our hypothesis is that in humans as in rats, the pheromones exuded by a male may be able to bring about a later age at menopause by increasing the likelihood of regular menstrual cycles of about twenty-nine days in length (Cutler et al. 1986). The longitudinal Tremin Research data, discussed in Chapter Three, showed that women with regular menstrual cycles of twenty-six to thirty-two days in length experienced a later age at menopause (Whelan et al. 1990).

Rural–Urban

In Mexico, Beyene (1986) reported a mean age of forty-two years at menopause among the rural Maya women in Chichimilá, Yucatán ($n = 71$). A slightly later mean of forty-four years was computed in two semi-rural towns, also in Yucatán (Canto-de-Cetina, Canto-Cetina, and Polanco-Reyes 1988). In and around the urban center of Progreso, Yucatán, Dickinson et al. (1992) found a mean age of 44.3 years at menopause. In the urban environment of Mexico City, investigators reported means of forty-five years (Parra-Cabrera et al. 1996) and 46.5 years (Garrido-Latorre et al. 1996). In the city of León, median ages at menopause were reported to be 48.2 (Garcia Vela, Nava, and Malacara 1987) and 48.5 (Velasco et al. 1990). This continuum, all within one country, suggests that women in urban areas experience a later age at menopause compared with women in rural areas, but, again, the differences can also be explained by the methods used to compute the average ages at menopause.

As another example, it is difficult to know whether women have an earlier or later age at menopause in urban Coimbra, Portugal, compared with rural Ança. Using retrospective ages at menopause among all women sampled, ages thirty-eight to ninety-one at interview, urban women recalled a later mean age at natural menopause (49.2 versus 48.2 years). However, using a status quo technique on a smaller sample of women, aged forty to sixty, urban women demonstrated an earlier median age at menopause (47.0 versus 48.5 years) (Guedes Pinto da Cunha 1984). In Finland, urban women have a slightly later age at menopause, but education is more important than place of residence (Luoto, Kaprio, and Uutela 1994).

Smoking Habits

Smoking has consistently been identified with an earlier age at menopause (Brambilla and McKinlay 1989; Do et al. 1998; Elias et al. 2003; Luoto, Kaprio, and Uutela 1994; Parazzini, Negri, and La Vecchia 1992; Reyes Cañizales et al. 2005; Reynolds and Obermeyer 2005; Shinberg 1998). Cramer and Xu (1996) showed that risk for an early menopause was most apparent for women who began smoking in their teens and that the risk for an early menopause increased progressively, in a dose-dependent way, with the number of pack-years of smoking. In Puebla, smoking before menopause resulted in an earlier age at menopause (Sievert and Hautaniemi 2003). In contrast, another study carried out in Mexico reported no association between age at menopause and smoking habits—"due to the low tobacco consumption found in this population" (Garrido-Latorre et al. 1996).

The finding that smokers experienced a dose-dependent decrease in age at menopause (Jick, Parker, and Morrison 1977) led Donald Mattison and colleagues to show that benzo(a)pyrene (a component of the tar fraction in cigarette smoke) and its metabolites reduced the fertility of female mice in a dose-dependent way. Later experiments demonstrated that mice treated with benzo(a)pyrene produced fewer corpora lutea and therefore were experiencing fewer ovulations. Mice also showed a dose-dependent decrease in oocyte number with a concomitant reduction in the reproductive lifespan (Mattison and Thomford 1987; Mattison and Thorgeirsson 1978).

In addition to reducing oocyte number, smoking has antiestrogenic effects, meaning that smoking causes estrogen levels to fall, through an effect on either estrogen production or estrogen metabolism. For example, smoking appears to alter estrogen-producing enzymes (Mattison and Thomford 1987). Smoking also exerts effects at the level of the hypothalamus and pituitary. The hypothalamus is rich in nicotine receptors, and smoking enhances dopamine production. Dopamine inhibits the secretion of gonadotrophic releasing hormone, which would ultimately affect estrogen production (Baron and Greenberg 1987). Parazzini,

Negri, and La Vecchia (1992) point out that ex-smokers have comparable ages at menopause compared with never-smokers, suggesting that the hormonal effect of smoking on risk of early menopause is short-term.

Alcohol

Compared with the interest in smoking, few studies have examined the consumption of alcohol in relation to age at menopause. Alcohol consumption increases levels of plasma estradiol in pre- and postmenopausal women (for a review of these studies see Gill 2000), and studies with very small sample sizes have shown that chronic alcohol abuse is associated with an earlier age at menopause (Gavaler 1985). One prospective postal survey carried out in the United Kingdom found that the onset of menopause appears to be later among women who consume alcohol in moderation. Moderation was defined as more than zero but less than seven drinks per week (Torgerson et al. 1994, 1997).

Age at Menarche

Conventional wisdom to the contrary, most studies have found no association between age at menarche and age at menopause (Guedes Pinto da Cunha 1984; Neri et al. 1982; Parazzini, Negri, and La Vecchia 1992; Stanford et al. 1987; Treloar 1974; van Noord et al. 1997; Whelan et al. 1990) within populations. In Puebla, neither menarche before age eleven nor menarche after age fourteen had significant effects on age at menopause compared with menarche at more usual ages (Sievert and Hautaniemi 2003).

Studies that have found an association are somewhat conflicting. For example, Cramer and Xu (1996) reported that an early age at menarche (less than twelve years) increased the risk of an early menopause (early menarche, early menopause). Ages at menarche and menopause were positively associated in Sweden (Rodstrom et al. 2003). Similarly, in the Netherlands, a later age at menarche was associated with a later age at menopause (Elias et al. 2003), although an earlier paper had reported no association (using a subset of the final study population, van Noord et al. 1997). On the other hand, Do et al. (1998), in a study of Australian twins, found that menarche later than age fourteen reduced the age at menopause (late menarche, early menopause). This association was also found among first-generation Mexican immigrants (Leidy 1998) and among the Blackfeet of Montana (Johnston 2001).

From a lifespan perspective, ages at menarche and menopause would *not* be expected to be consistently associated across populations, because menarche occurs after only a little more than a decade of life. On the other hand, menopause occurs after four or five decades of living—time enough for the two events to become completely dissociated.

Menstrual Cycle Characteristics

Using Treloar's longitudinal data set, Whelan et al. (1990) found that women who had a short menstrual cycle (an average cycle length of less than twenty-six days) when they were twenty to thirty-five years of age had an earlier age at menopause compared with women who had a median cycle length of twenty-six to thirty-two days. Women who experienced long cycles (an average cycle length of thirty-three days or longer) were more likely to have late ages at menopause. Cramer and Xu (1996) also found that short cycles were associated with an earlier age at menopause.

Stanford et al. (1987) looked at whether or not menstrual periods were regular or irregular during the early reproductive years (before age twenty-five or first live birth). They found that women who reported regular menstrual periods early on experienced an earlier menopause compared with women who reported irregular periods. On the other hand, Parazzini, Negri, and La Vecchia (1992) and Reynolds and Obermeyer (2005) reported no association with regularity of periods.

Some investigators have argued that short cycles or regular cycles are associated with an earlier age at menopause because women ovulate more often. As noted earlier, however, ovulation has little effect on the rate of loss of ovarian follicles (and ultimately on age at menopause). As discussed in Chapters One and Two, almost all follicle loss occurs through the process of atresia (degeneration). It may be that short cycles or regular cycles are indicative of hormonal imbalances that increase the rate of follicular atresia across the lifespan.

Use of Hormonal Birth Control

There is no association between the use of hormonal birth control and age at menopause in studies carried out in Massachusetts, Mexico, and Spain (Brambilla and McKinlay 1989; Reynolds and Obermeyer 2005; Sievert and Hautaniemi 2003). Stanford et al. (1987) found that women who used hormonal birth control experienced a later age at menopause, but this relationship no longer existed after controlling for the duration of oral contraceptive use. Among the Blackfeet of Montana, women who ever used oral contraceptives experienced menopause 5.5 years later than did women who never used oral contraceptives (Johnston 2001). In contrast, Garrido-Latorre et al. (1996) found an earlier age at menopause among contraceptive users in Mexico City.

Reproductive History

Consistent across studies is the finding that women who have never given birth (nulliparous) have an earlier age at menopause compared with women who have given birth (Cramer and Xu 1996; Do et al. 1998; Elias et al. 2003; Parazzini, Negri, and La Vecchia 1992; Sievert and Hautaniemi 2003; Whelan et al. 1990). Some investigators have also found a later menopause with an increasing number of pregnancies (Garrido-Latorre et al. 1996; Stanford et al. 1987) or a trend toward a later menopause with increasing numbers of pregnancies (Cramer and Xu 1996; Parazzini, Negri, and La Vecchia 1992). For example, Whelan et al. (1990) found that age at menopause increased from 50.0 years among women with no children to 50.5 (one to two children) to 50.7 (three to four children) to 51.0 among women with five or more children. These researchers double-checked their data by restricting the analysis to only women whose last birth was before age forty (to be sure that the trend was not because women with a later age at menopause *could* have more children). The trend remained. Other investigators have found no association between number of children and age at menopause (McKinlay et al. 1992; Shinberg 1998).

Best Models and Cross-Population Comparisons

Investigators try to come up with the "best" model to explain variation in age at menopause for their particular populations of study. For example, in Puebla, the largest effect on age at menopause was from smoking. Smokers had about an 85 percent greater risk of menopause across time, and therefore a lower age at menopause, compared with nonsmokers. Never having been pregnant raised the risk by 65 percent, and lowered the age at menopause. Similarly, a higher BMI at age eighteen lowered the age at menopause. Only more years of education reduced the risk of menopause across time (and raised age at menopause), compared with women with little education, in the final model (Sievert and Hautaniemi 2003).

The final model put forth by Stanford et al. (1987) suggested that a greater number of live births, menstrual cycle irregularity, higher income, and higher levels of education postponed age at menopause. In Italy, the final model by Parazzini, Negri, and La Vecchia (1992) was made up of smoking and parity. In the United Kingdom, Torgerson et al. (1994) concluded that age at menopause was later among women who did not smoke, among women whose mothers experienced an older age at maternal menopause, and among women with more children, lower social class (based on husband's occupation), higher alcohol use, and higher meat consumption.

Because each group of researchers collects different variables, the final models differ. In addition, variables have culture-specific attributes that influence the explanatory models and can result in contrasting results across populations. For example, differing educational opportunities for women result in different mean levels of education, so that education categories (low, medium, high) must differ. In Mexico and Italy, low education is best described as zero to six years, whereas in the United Sates less than twelve years is considered low. Torgerson et al. (1994) collected social class data (I–V) rather than education level. Cultural characteristics influence smoking habits, number of children, and variation in income. In addition, as discussed earlier, there is probably a strong genetic component to age at menopause so that some degree of cross-population difference is explained by variation in genetic constraints.

CHAPTER FIVE

The Discomforts of Menopause

[The discovery of unexpected symptoms] does not mean that such patients are not conveying valid information about their experience of bodily processes; it only demonstrates a gap between experience and biology. Social expectation, cultural priority, and personal response fill that gap.

Arthur Kleinman, *Writing at the Margin* (1995)

Like the wide range in variation in age at menopause, a wide range of variation in discomforts or symptoms is associated with the menopause transition. Table 5.1 shows some of the symptom frequencies reported during the two weeks before interview in western Massachusetts; Puebla, Mexico; and Asunción, Paraguay. In western Massachusetts, 22 percent of women reported hot flashes (Leidy 1997) compared with 50 percent in Puebla and 43 percent in Asunción.

TABLE 5.1

Percentage of Women of Menopausal Age Reporting Discomforts

Symptoms	Western Massachusetts (n = 155)	Puebla, Mexico (n = 755)	Asunción, Paraguay (n = 505)
Lack of energy	63	70	73
Aches/stiffness in joints	62	56	71
Nervous tension	50	66	77
Trouble sleeping	48	52	45
Headaches	42	53	79
Hot flashes	22	50	43

Source: Leidy (1997); Sievert (2001a); unpublished data.

The most commonly reported symptoms in Massachusetts were lack of energy and stiffness/aches in the joints; in Puebla the most common symptoms were lack of energy and nervous tension; in Asunción the most common were headaches and nervous tension. How can we understand variation in symptom frequencies reported within and across populations? As noted in Chapter Three, cross-cultural comparisons of symptoms at menopause are valuable for understanding many aspects of women's health and well-being.

What Are the Discomforts?

Table 5.2 lists the top four complaints reported by women of menopausal age (age ranges at interview were all within thirty-five to sixty-five years) in twenty-four studies of current symptoms or symptoms experienced during the two or four weeks prior to interview. As can be seen in the table, only six of the twenty-four populations identified hot flashes or night sweats (in italic) as one of the top four complaints.

Of the complaints in table 5.2, the most common is headache, followed by joint pain/stiffness, irritability, lack of energy, and nervous tension. If backache is combined with joint pain/stiffness, then the broad category of muscular-skeletal-joint complaints tops the list. Eight of the studies in table 5.2 did not include somatic complaints in their symptom lists, therefore women could only indicate the presence or absence of vasomotor (for example, hot flashes) or psychological symptoms (Agoestina and van Keep 1984; Boulet et al. 1994). In Bangkok, numbness in the extremities was the only somatic complaint assessed (Sukwatana et al. 1991). Thus of the twenty-four studies cited in table 5.2, only fifteen asked about somatic symptoms. Of those fifteen, thirteen studies identified muscular-skeletal-joint pain or stiffness as one of the top four complaints. Only studies in Lebanon (Obermeyer, Ghorayeb, and Reynolds 1999) and the United Kingdom (Thompson, Hart, and Durno 1973) did not find muscular-skeletal-joint complaints at the top of their frequency lists.

Although it has been well established that the only symptoms associated with declining estrogen levels are vasomotor symptoms and vaginal dryness (WHO 1981), it is clear that women aged thirty-five to sixty-five, in sixteen different countries, have other complaints. As Oldenhave et al. (1993) point out, hot flashes are relatively easy to cope with because they are short-lived and occur infrequently in most women. Instead, many women are bothered to a greater extent by the "atypical" complaints, such as bone pain or depression— "complaints for which they often do not have an explanation and for which they seek medical care" (779). Here I focus on four discomforts experienced by some women of menopausal age and attributed to menopause by health care providers: somatic complaints (muscular-skeletal-joint pain/stiffness), psychological complaints (depression), vaginal dryness, and a decreased desire for sex.

TABLE 5.2

Top Four Complaints Reported by Women of Menopausal Age

Country	Sites or Groups	Most Frequent Complaint	Second	Third	Fourth	Source
Australia	Brisbane	Dry skin	Backache	Forgetfulness	Problems sleeping	O'Connor et al. (1995)
	Melbourne	Aches/stiff joints	Lack of energy	Nervous tension	Backaches	Dennerstein et al. (1993)
Canada	Manitoba	Lack of energy	Headaches	Aches/stiff joints	Hot flashes	Avis et al. (1993)
Finland	Helsinki	Tiredness	Hot flashes	Backache	Headache	Hemminki, Topo, and Kangas (1995)
Hong Kong	Five cities	Headache	Dizziness	Irritability	Depression	Boulet et al. (1994)
Indonesia		Headache	Dizziness	Irritability	Insomnia	Boulet et al. (1994)
	Bandung	Headache	Vertigo	Insomnia	Palpitations	Agoestina and van Keep (1984)
Japan	Kobe, Kyoto, Nagano	Shoulder stiffness	Headache	Lumbago	Constipation	Lock (1993)
Korea	Seoul	Palpitations	Dizziness	Headache	Hot flashes	Boulet et al. (1994)
Lebanon	Beirut	Fatigue/weakness	Impatience/ nervousness	Anxiety	Memory loss	Obermeyer, Ghorayeb, and Reynolds (1999)
Malaysia		Headache	Hot flashes	Depression	Palpitations	Boulet et al. (1994)
Mexico	Puebla	Lack of energy	Nervousness	Back pain	Joint aches/stiffness	Sievert (2001a)

(continued)

TABLE 5.2

Top Four Complaints Reported by Women of Menopausal Age *(continued)*

Country	Sites or Groups	Most Frequent Complaint	Second	Third	Fourth	Source
Philippines	Manila	Headache	Irritability	Anxiety	Dizziness	Boulet et al. (1994)
Singapore		Headache	Irritability	Anxiety	Insomnia	Boulet et al. (1994)
Taiwan		Headache	Anxiety	Irritability	Insomnia	Boulet et al. (1994)
Thailand	Bangkok	Dizziness	Tiredness	Joint aches	Irritability	Punyahotra, Dennerstein, and Lehert (1997)
	Bangkok	*Hot flashes*	Heat intolerance	Numbness of extremities	Palpitation	Sukwatana et al. (1991)
UK	Aberdeen	Depression	Tiredness	Headaches	*Night sweats*	Thompson, Hart, and Durno (1973)
U.S.	Mass.	Aches/stiff joints	Lack of energy	Headaches	Feeling blue/ depressed	Avis et al. (1993)
U.S. SWAN	African-Am.	Stiffness	Irritable	Tense	Headache	Avis et al. (2001)
	Hispanic	Tense	Headache	Depressed	Stiffness	
	Chinese	Stiffness	Irritable	Tense	Headache	
	Japanese	Stiffness	Irritable	Headache	Tense	
	White	Tense	Irritable	Stiffness	Headache	

Muscle-Joint-Bone Pain/Stiffness

In answer to the open-ended question "what symptom(s) do you associate with the menopause transition," one of the first participants in the menopause study in Puebla, Mexico, answered "dolores de huesos" or bone pain. This answer caught me by surprise, because I was poised to write "bochornos" or hot flashes, as I would have written in western Massachusetts or Slovenia. Instead, this participant, a domestic worker who cleaned houses and cooked for middle-class families, directed my attention to one of the most common complaints expressed by women of menopausal age.

The symptom frequencies in table 5.1 summarize responses to structured, closed question lists. For example, in Puebla, we used the Everyday Complaints symptom list, structured questions that asked whether or not a woman had experienced a particular symptom within the past two weeks. Of the 775 respondents, 55.6 percent reported joint aches/stiffness and 55.8 percent reported back pain (Sievert and Goode-Null 2005). These frequencies were slightly higher than the percentage of women reporting hot flashes (49.6 percent). We also asked an open-ended question, what symptoms do you associate with the end of menstruation? The most common answers to this question were hot flashes (52.8 percent), bone pain (46.7 percent), headaches (45.3 percent), irritability (42.8 percent), depression (9.6 percent), and hemorrhage (6.5 percent).

When I returned from Mexico, I reexamined other studies of complaints reported by women of menopausal age and found that bone pain, or muscular-skeletal-joint pain/stiffness, was surprisingly common. For example, during the two weeks prior to interview, more Australian women aged forty-five to fifty-five reported backaches (36.7 percent) and aches or stiff joints (48.8 percent) than hot flashes (28 percent) (Dennerstein et al. 1993). This finding in Melbourne held consistent in Brisbane, Australia, where 49 percent of 381 women aged forty-five to fifty-four reported backaches in the two weeks prior to interview, but only 25 percent reported hot flashes (O'Connor et al. 1995). In Japan, more women aged forty-five to fifty-five reported back pain (24 percent) and joint pain (15 percent) than hot flashes (12 percent) during the two weeks before interview (Lock 1993). Japanese Americans in Los Angeles also reported more stiffness (50 percent) than hot flashes (12 percent) (Avis et al. 2001). As a final example, more women aged forty to fifty-nine reported back pain (53 percent) and joint pain (55 percent) than hot flashes (27 percent) during the two weeks prior to interview in Bangkok, Thailand (Punyahotra, Dennerstein, and Lehert 1997).

Musculo-skeletal complaints are particularly frequent among women drawn from patient populations (Kirchengast 1993; Rizk et al. 1998). For example, in Turkey, muscle-joint-bone pain was the most common complaint, reported among 82 percent of women at a menopause clinic (Carda et al. 1998). It may be that women suffering from "atypical" muscular-skeletal-joint complaints are more likely to see physicians for help during the menopausal years (Oldenhave et al. 1993). A comparison with males in this age range would be valuable to determine whether the symptoms are more common among menopausal women.

The symptoms may simply reflect the general aches associated with aging (Bradsher and McKinlay 2000). For instance, in the menopause clinic in Turkey, "muscle-joint-bone pain" was the symptom most often associated with menopause (Carda et al. 1998), but participant ages ranged from forty to seventy. In a small study of menopause in the mountains of Slovenia, we found that 59 percent of women aged thirty-two to eighty-five years reported back pain and 53 percent reported joint aches, but only 24 percent reported hot flashes during the two weeks prior to interview (Sievert et al. 2004).

Samples drawn from clinical populations and samples with broad age ranges are problematic; nevertheless, there is enough evidence from general-population-based surveys of women aged forty-five to fifty-five to conclude that menopausal women do experience musculo-skeletal-joint complaints, often with a greater frequency than hot flashes. A biocultural perspective can contribute to a better understanding of musculo-skeletal-joint complaints associated with the menopause transition.

Musculoskeletal symptoms in women of menopausal age may be related to hormonal changes; however, the role of declining estrogen levels with menopause in the etiology of osteoarthritis is unclear, because treatment with estrogen has conflicting effects on cartilage degradation and repair (Birchfield 2001). Cartilage cells have estrogen receptors; however, the effect of estrogen on bone may be of greater importance (Felson and Nevitt 1999). Women taking HT have demonstrated both lower (Felson and Nevitt 1999; Nevitt et al. 1996) and higher prevalences of osteoarthritis (Von Mühlen et al. 2002).

Risk factors associated with the development of osteoarthritis include excessive body weight (Birchfield 2001; Gold et al. 2000; Spence 1989) and strenuous, repetitive exercise (Birchfield 2001). As the epidemic of obesity continues, the complaint of joint pain may occur more frequently in future cohorts of women reaching menopausal age. With regard to exercise, a survey of women's roles cross-culturally demonstrates that many individuals perform repetitive tasks that require kneeling, crouching, and walking long distances. On the other hand, a lack of exercise can also be detrimental to skeletal/joint health (Birchfield 2001; Gold et al. 2000).

Although there is considerable variation in the type of pain and/or stiffness reported across cultures, the broader prevalence of muscular-skeletal-joint complaints among women of menopausal age is not known, because the relevant questions often are not asked (see table 6.2). For example, the seven East Asian studies compiled by Boulet et al. (1994) were carried out by the International Health Foundation in 1989 "in an attempt to ascertain whether the climacteric as a concept existed in south-east Asian countries and to what extent it was recognized as such" (Boulet et al. 1994:158). Only vasomotor and psychological symptoms were included on the symptom list. The same was true for studies carried out in Indonesia (Agoestina and van Keep 1984), California (von Mühlen, Kritz-Siverstein, and Barrett-Conner 1995), Bangkok (Chaikittisilpa et al. 1997), and Sweden (Hammar et al. 1984).

In summary, "bone pain" appears to be more common among women of menopausal age than might be expected. The extent of musculo-skeletal-joint complaints across cultures is not known, however, because of the broad age ranges sampled (unlike hot flashes, osteoarthritis increases with postmenopausal age) and the omission of somatic discomforts from symptom lists. The extent to which musculo-skeletal-joint complaints are caused by the hormonal fluctuations of the menopause transition or by the lifelong activity patterns of women laboring at home, in factories, or in fields is not known.

Depression

Whereas musculo-skeletal-joint pain or stiffness has seldom been the exclusive subject of investigation in studies of menopause, depression has a long history of association with the shift from the reproductive to the nonreproductive phase of life (C. B. Ballinger 1990; Rosenthal 1974). In 1896 Emil Kraepelin classified involutional melancholia as depression occurring for the first time among women after menopause (ages forty to fifty-five) and among men in late middle age (fifty to sixty-five). "Involutional" is a general term that refers to a gradual and progressive decline in any tissue or organ function. In the case of involutional melancholia, "involutional" referred more specifically to the decline in reproductive function. Kraepelin speculated that involutional melancholia was caused by external stress and was characterized by anxious depression, apprehension, and delusions (H. Ford 1975). The prognosis was poor, and the course of the disease was prolonged. In a study of patients hospitalized for involutional melancholia between 1930 and 1939 at Iowa Psychopathic Hospital, only 46 percent recovered over an average of forty-nine months, 18 percent did not recover, and 36 percent died. At the time, therapy emphasized bed rest, nutrition, isolation from the family, and prevention of suicide (Rosenthal 1974).

Depression was not limited to Iowa. In an often-quoted selection from the Human Relations Area Files files, menopause was believed to induce insanity among the rural Irish: "In order to ward off this condition, some women have retired from life in their mid-forties and, in a few cases, have confined themselves to bed until death, years later. . . .the harbingers of 'insanity' are simply the physical symptoms announcing the onset of menopause. In Inis Beag, these include severe headaches, hot flashes, faintness in crowds and enclosed places, and severe anxiety" (Messenger 1971:15). Messenger and his wife carried out their fieldwork among the rural Irish between 1958 and 1966, not long after the American Psychiatric Association published its first Diagnostic and Statistical Manual, Mental Disorders (DSM-I) in 1952.

In the DSM-I involutional melancholia, or involutional psychotic reaction, was listed under the subheading of "disorders due to disturbances of metabolism, growth, nutrition, or endocrine function" (H. Ford 1975). This classification portrayed involutional melancholia as a distinct disease entity; it also reflected an understanding of the endocrine changes that accompany menopause. Estrogens had been isolated at the beginning of the century (Tepperman and Tepperman 1987) and this "internal secretion," lasting throughout a woman's life, was thought to consist of "various chemical substances, (with) a tremendous influence not only on the development of the woman's body, but also on her feelings" (Robinson 1938:14). This secretion was thought to be responsible not only for female secondary sexual characteristics but for sexual health, general well-being, energy, and mental alertness as well (C. B. Ballinger 1990).

Although there was general agreement during the first half of the twentieth century that involutional melancholia was a specific type of depression experienced by both women and men (but primarily women), opinions varied as to exactly what caused the symptoms. Some authors (such as Robinson) attributed depression to estrogen deficiency. Psychoanalysts, such as Freud, Helene Deutsch, and Therese Benedek, compared the climacteric to the storms of adolescence (Delaney, Lupton, and Toth 1988; Lock 1993; Scarf 1980). In 1950 Fessler theorized that "to a woman the ability to have a child is her compensation for not having a penis. Menstruation is the constant reminder of this and is thus a penis substitute and implies female completeness. The cessation of menses therefore may cause regression and penis envy" (in Rosenthal 1974:704).

Through the late 1950s and 1960s, psychology textbooks began to include more sociocultural aspects of the involutional period, such as role loss and shifts in identity (C. B. Ballinger 1990; Rosenthal 1974). An interesting cross-cultural study during this time was an analysis of Zulu dreaming. Lee (1958) collected the obstetric history of over four hundred women to demonstrate that young married women dreamt more often of babies, reflecting the intense social pressure they felt to prove their fertility. In contrast, older married women experienced nightmares of flooded rivers. These dreams were interpreted by Lee as representing fear of further deliveries in conflict with social pressure to continue bearing children for as long as possible. This nightmare was experienced by women through the menopause transition, as there continued to be "conflict between the motives conditioned by years of social pressure [to continue bearing children] and the new-found status of 'a man' granted by the society" (Lee 1958:277). According to Lee, dreams are "circumscribed and influenced by the social pressures and sanctions of the culture" (266). Lee interpreted these dreams to be caused by role conflict, not estrogen decline.

Another cross-cultural example comes from Field (1962), who examined rural cases of mental illness among the Ashanti people who visited religious shrines. Field noted that, in general, "in rural Ghana, Involutional Depression with agitation is, as in our own society, one of the commonest and most clearly defined of mental illnesses" (1962:149). The patients so labeled were women who "launched a fleet of well-brought up children" and then felt useless. Additionally distressing was the culturally sanctioned practice of husbands taking extra, younger wives to continue bearing children. "Most women . . . are worried by these social hazards of the menopause, and many of them, when they first become aware of amenorrhea, go from shrine to shrine over several years with the plaint, 'I am pregnant, but the pregnancy doesn't grow'" (150).

Ashanti women suffering from involutional depression, according to Field, exhibited all of the symptoms in the DSM description, such as worry, anxiety, agitation, severe insomnia, feelings of guilt, somatic preoccupations, and delusions. In this case the fieldwork (1955–1958) was carried out when the diagnosis of involutional melancholia was commonly applied in Western psychiatry.

When the DSM-II was published in 1968, bringing American psychiatric practices closer to the World Health Organization International Classification of Diseases, involutional melancholia was classified under "affective psychoses" (H. Ford 1975). The description of the illness, however, indicated uncertainty over whether the practitioner was actually able to differentiate between involutional melancholia and other depressive syndromes: "Involutional melancholia is a disorder occurring in the involutional period and characterized by worry, anxiety, agitation, and severe insomnia. Feelings of guilt and somatic preoccupations are frequently present and may be of delusional proportions. . . . [It is] recommended that involutional patients not be given this diagnosis unless all other affective disorders have been ruled out" (DSM-II 1968:36).

The behavioral pictures for both the reactive and the involutional depressions were identical. The choice of diagnosis was determined only by the age of the woman and/or her menopausal status. Menopause was stereotyped as the dominant factor in the midlife of women, so that when a patient presented symptoms of depression, there was "a tendency to focus automatically on the menstrual history, as if it [would] explain the symptomatology of the patient" (Notman 1980:95).

When the DSM-III was published in 1979, the illness category of involutional melancholia was no longer included, although the debate over the connection between menopause and depression persists. As C. B. Ballinger (1990) points out, "the psychiatrists see many women with psychiatric disorders, only a few of whom are menopausal, while the gynecologists see many menopausal women of whom a large number present with psychiatric symptoms" (755). Some authorities continue to defend the estrogen connection to psychological symptoms, in part on the basis of the consistent finding that rates of depression are higher in women than in men (Weissman 1979; Weissman and Olfson 1995). However, there is no direct association between hormones and mood (Ballinger et al. 1987; M. S. Hunter 1990; Spinelli 2000).

There is evidence that estrogen modulates the synthesis of central nervous system enzymes, peptides, neurotransmitters, and receptors. Estrogen increases norepinephrine availability through the inhibition of monoamine oxidase and increases serotonin uptake through its effect on serotonin receptors (reviewed by Spinelli 2000). Evidence for the mood-enhancing effects of HT is inconsistent, however, leading Spinelli (2000), Pearlstein (1995), and M. S. Hunter (1994) to conclude that estrogen appears to improve mood in healthy women, but appears to be ineffective as a treatment for women with major depression. Progesterone, as a component of HT, may promote depression (Pearlstein 1995; Sherwin 1991) by decreasing norepinephrine concentrations.

The majority of menopausal women do not show signs of depression or other psychological symptoms (Bradsher and McKinlay 2000), and most scientists now argue that the frequency of psychiatric symptoms is no higher for menopausal women than for women in other age groups (Gath and Isles 1990; Matthews et al. 1990; Obermeyer, Ghorayeb, and Reynolds 2000; Rannevik et al. 1995; Weissman 1979; Weissman and Olfson 1995). However, factor analytic studies of menopausal symptoms often statistically extract psychological symptoms as the first symptom cluster (Collins and Landgren 1994; Dennerstein et al. 1993; Kaufert and Syrotuik 1981; Greene 1976; Holte and Mikkelsen 1991b; von Mühlen et al. 1995). In addition, peri- or postmenopausal women report significantly ($p < .05$) more psychological symptoms compared with premenopausal women in cross-sectional studies in Australia (O'Connor et al. 1995), England (M. S. Hunter 1990), Thailand (Punyahotra, Dennerstein, and Lehert 1997), Hong Kong and Malaysia (Boulet et al. 1994).[1]

In a number of studies, women reporting psychological complaints were more likely to have consulted their physicians about menopause compared with women who reported hot flashes (S. E. Ballinger 1985; Boulet et al. 1994). Consistent with the epigraph that begins this chapter, Boulet and colleagues suggest that psychological symptoms could be "essentially a means of communication," that "vasomotor distress might, in some way or another, be 'translated' into psychological distress in south-east Asia" (Boulet et al. 1994:172). Alternatively, menopause can offer a socially legitimate reason for symptoms that might otherwise be labeled neurotic (S. E. Ballinger 1985; C. B. Ballinger 1990).

The percentage of women from the Norwegian Menopause Project who reported "frequent" mood swings, irritability, or weepiness in relation to menopausal status is shown in figure 5.1. This project, carried out in Oslo, Norway, recruited 1,886 participants aged forty-five to fifty-five from the population registry. Women were classified as premenopausal ("cycling") if they reported regular menstrual cycles and had menstruated within the past two months.

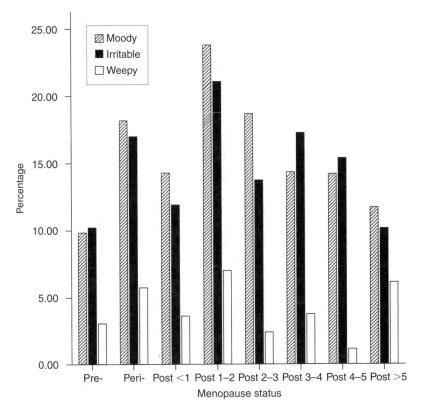

FIGURE 5.1 The percentage of women who reported "frequent" mood swings, irritability, or weepiness in relation to menopausal status, the Norwegian Menopause Project. Postmenopausal subjects were classified into six categories: those who had not menstruated for six to twelve months (post <1), for one to two years (post 1–2), for two to three years (post 2–3), for three to four years (post 3–4), for four to five years (post 4–5), or for more than five years (post >6).

Data drawn from Holte (1991).

Perimenopause was defined as having irregular periods or as having ceased menstruation within the past two to six months. Postmenopausal subjects were classified into six categories based on time since final menstruation. As figure 5.1 shows, women who were one to two years postmenopausal reported the highest frequency of symptoms; however, the differences were only significant across all categories for weepiness ($p < .01$) (Holte 1991).

Researchers studying the longitudinal data from the Massachusetts Women's Health Study found that experiencing a long perimenopausal period (at least twenty-seven months) was associated with a slightly increased risk of depression (Avis et al. 1994). The study also demonstrated that depression associated with the perimenopausal state "is *transitory;* as women become postmenopausal, their rates of depression decline" (217, emphasis in original). The increased risk of depression during the perimenopause is partly explained by symptom frequencies—women who reported hot flashes, night sweats, or menstrual problems had higher rates of depression.

Although an argument can be made for an ovarian etiology for depressed mood at menopause, it is important to remember that, from a biocultural perspective, changing biology is just one aspect of midlife. For example, depressed mood during menopause can be predicted by past depressive episodes associated with oral contraceptive use, premenstrual time periods, and postpartum periods (Avis et al. 1994; S. E. Ballinger 1985; M. S. Hunter 1990; Stewart and Boydell 1993). It may be that some women experience increased sensitivity to normal hormonal changes (Stewart and Boydell 1993). Alternatively, mood changes may be due to loss of sleep because of hot flashes (Hammar et al. 1984) or due to changes in family relationships during this period of the lifespan (Kaufert, Gilbert, and Tate 1992; McKinlay, McKinlay and Brambilla 1987; Scarf 1980; Uphold and Susman 1981).

Many potential problems confront midlife women in all countries, including marital stresses (Finkler 1994), adolescent rebellion, children leaving home (or returning), and physical illness of self, partner, or parents (Dennerstein 1996). A number of studies have found that psychosocial factors (Hunter, Battersby, and Whitehead 1986; McKinlay, McKinlay, and Brambilla 1987) and coping skills (S. E. Ballinger 1985) account for more of the variation in depressed mood than do the hormonal changes of menopause.

In a longitudinal study of menopause in England, M. S. Hunter (1990) found that the experience of stress before menopause, hypochondriacal concerns, and not exercising on a regular basis were factors associated with depression when women became menopausal. In addition, women who held negative beliefs about menopause were also more likely to become depressed. "Negative beliefs could act as a filter through which physiological and emotional sensations are experienced, thus influencing women's perceptions and interpretations of the menopause" (M. S. Hunter 1990:364). In Manitoba, women who saw their health as poor were seventeen times more likely to be depressed than women in good health. The likelihood of depression also increased if women were stressed by their relationships with their husbands and children but, interestingly, the relative odds for depression were not affected by children's leaving home (Kaufert, Gilbert, and Tate 1992).

In conclusion, a biocultural approach to depression suggests that, although estrogen is involved in the modulation of neurotransmitters that may affect mood, many midlife women throughout the world today are annoyed by persistent hot flashes, concerned about adolescent children, responsible for aging parents, working inside and outside of the home, and tangled in marriage to midlife men. Cultural contexts provide unique pressures and concerns that contribute to the risk of depression among women of menopausal age.

Vaginal Dryness

When I first started to study menopause in my midtwenties, I mentioned my interest to a saleswoman in upstate New York while shopping for a suit for a conference. She surprised me by following me into the dressing room and asking, in a whisper, what to do about vaginal dryness. The question no longer surprises me. Although hot flashes grab the spotlight, I am often quietly asked about vaginal dryness. Perhaps relatedly, I am also asked whether a woman's desire for sex increases or decreases at menopause. As noted in Chapter Three, whether or not older women were sexually active was often the only question asked about menopause by male anthropologists during the early years of ethnographic inquiry.

The issues of vaginal dryness and changes in interest in sex overlap, because vaginal dryness can cause sex to be painful (a condition called dyspareunia). On the other hand, as will be described, changes in sexual desire are more complicated than vaginal dryness.

While hot flashes will eventually diminish and even cease with time, vulvovaginal atrophy (deterioration) will only worsen. The vagina and vulva (the exterior tissue around the vagina) are rich in estrogen receptors,[2] and as estrogen levels continue to decline after menopause (figure 2.4), the receptors receive less and less estrogen, leading to a loss of elasticity, vascularity (blood supply), and adiposity (fat) in these regions (Bachmann and Nevadunsky 2000). Women who undergo menopause by hysterectomy with both ovaries removed often have the worst trouble with vaginal dryness, because of the sudden loss of estrogen, changes in blood and nerve supply, and changes to the vaginal vault (the shape is modified by the removal of the uterus and sometimes the cervix). Women who are having sexual relations sometimes experience pain and postcoital bleeding. Women who are not having sexual relations do not necessarily notice a decline in vaginal moistness; however, the decline in vaginal lubrication can lead to irritation, burning sensations, and more urinary tract infections as the normal vaginal flora changes (Priestley et al. 1997). The vaginal flora changes because the vaginal pH becomes more alkaline (a pH of 3.8 to 4.2 is normal).

Topical estrogen (meaning estrogen that is applied to just the affected tissues) reverses atrophic changes, but some women prefer over-the-counter lubricants and moisturizers. In Mexico, women tell me that they use cooking oil or hand lotion to reduce vaginal dryness during sex. Continued sexual activity can also help to reduce vaginal dryness.

In Australia, Dennerstein et al. (2000) found an increase in the frequency of vaginal dryness from less than 5 percent of women during the early perimenopause to more than 20 percent of women during the first year after menopause to more than 40 percent of women at three years postmenopause.

The researchers observed that it was not age but the reduction in circulating estrogens that was associated with genital atrophy. In Puebla, Mexico, we found that women with hysterectomies and natural menopause were significantly more likely to report vaginal dryness (30 percent and 28 percent, respectively) compared with premenopausal women (13 percent, $p < .01$).

As shown in table 5.3, no women in Asunción, Paraguay, described their vaginal dryness to be "extreme" *(intensamente)*, but women who experienced menopause naturally or by hysterectomy were more likely to qualify their vaginal dryness as "quite a bit" *(bastante)*. On the other hand, women did use the "extreme" category to classify their loss of sexual desire, as shown in table 5.4, and women who had undergone a natural menopause were most likely to report an extreme loss of sexual desire. This finding suggests that there is more to the loss of sexual desire than just vaginal dryness.

TABLE 5.3

Percentage of Women Reporting Vaginal Dryness in Asunción, Paraguay

Menopause Status	N	None	A Little	Quite a Bit	Extreme
Premenopausal	263	72%	25%	2%	0
Natural menopause	133	51	40	9	0
Posthysterectomy	61	57	33	10	0

Source: Unpublished data.

TABLE 5.4

Percentage of Women Reporting a Loss in Desire for Sex in Asunción, Paraguay

Menopause Status	N	None	A Little	Quite a Bit	Extreme
Premenopausal	251	41%	46%	12%	1%
Natural menopause	120	27	30	27	17
Posthysterectomy	52	52	23	13	12

Source: Unpublished data.

Changes in Sexual Desire

Some researchers argue that, similar to vaginal dryness, a loss of desire for sex has hormonal origins. In addition to a loss of estrogen and the accompanying decline in vaginal elasticity and moistness, ovarian aging is also associated with a loss of androgens (for example, testosterone). Androgens are produced by the ovarian stroma (tissue that fills in between the ovarian follicles) (25 percent), the adrenal glands (25 percent), and by peripheral conversion (50 percent). The hormones that are converted peripherally come in equal amounts from the ovary and adrenal glands, so the removal of both ovaries removes 50 percent of the androgens normally produced in a woman's body (25 percent direct from the ovary, and 25 percent from the ovary but converted peripherally). In addition to a lack of genital response, the loss of androgen may also lead to loss of sexual thoughts and fantasies as well as the inability to respond to cues and triggers that would have elicited sexual desire in the past (Basson 2000).

There is however good evidence that, for women, sexual desire is much more complicated that simply a change in hormonal status. In the often-cited study of sexual dysfunction from the United States National Health and Social Life Survey, women aged fifty to fifty-nine were more likely to report trouble lubricating but *less* likely to report a lack of interest in sex compared with women aged eighteen to twenty-nine (Laumann, Paik, and Rosen 1999). However, women who reported low levels of general happiness were more than twice as likely to report low sexual desire and sexual pain, and more than five times as likely to report an arousal disorder (Laumann, Paik, and Rosen 1999). A similar pattern was demonstrated in relation to a woman's satisfaction with her primary partner.

Basson (2000) describes the major components of women's sexual satisfaction as including trust, intimacy, the ability to be vulnerable, respect, communication, and affection, as well as pleasure from sensual touching. She goes on to explain that a woman's motivation to participate in sexual activities may stem from rewards or gains that are not strictly sexual (for example, increased commitment and emotional closeness), and that sexual desire in women is a responsive rather than a spontaneous event. Important with regard to menopause, a pleasant physical experience is necessary to allow the sexual response to continue in the long term. Pain with intercourse due to vaginal dryness can thus reduce motivation and ultimately become associated with a general shutting down of sexual interest.

Variables that interfere with a woman's sexual interest include distractions (such as children), fatigue, and interpersonal issues (Basson 2000). As one fifty-seven-year-old women explained to me in Puebla, "el sexo ya no llama atención" (sex is no longer of interest). She wasn't sure if this was because of her hysterectomy, because she was so tired—caring for the house, her children, babysitting for her five-year-old grandchild—because of her age, or because sex hurt due to vaginal dryness. She went on to say that she didn't care what her husband did, "el puede ir con quien quiera" (he can go [have sex] with whoever he wants) because men still have sexual desires. For her, however, "todo está acabado" (it's all finished).

A forty-seven-year-old woman explained that her husband was always verbally abusive and wouldn't let her leave the house. Finally, with the excuse that sex hurt too much due to vaginal dryness, she refused all intimacy. Her husband now says that she is no better than a dog underfoot, but she still has no desire for sex with him. She wondered aloud whether her lack of desire was because of the hormonal changes or because she was so resentful of the way he had treated her for so many years.

Such stories are not unusual. These accounts from Puebla are very similar to those collected by Finkler (1994) in her study of women's pain in Mexico City. They illustrate that the lack of desire for sex has emotional roots far deeper than the withdrawal of estrogen from vaginal receptors. Treating these women with HT and a touch of testosterone will not fix the exhaustion and emotional heartbreak. When women in Puebla want to continue sexual relations with their partner, they use cooking oil or hand cream to counteract vaginal dryness. The biocultural perspective offers a holistic approach to better understand the complexities of symptom experience.

CHAPTER SIX

Hot Flashes

Clinically speaking, hot flashes are symptoms of menopause. But meno-pause is the cessation of a process, which means hot flashes are a mani-festation of *nothing*. I don't understand why *nothing* should have symptoms. Unlike menstrual periods, hot flashes serve no purpose such as the sloughing off of old tissue or new issue. Their heat cannot be har-nessed as energy for other purposes; like life, they are unpredictable, uncontrollable, uncomfortable and unfair.

B. Raskin, *Hot Flashes: The Novel* (1987)

In Barbara Raskin's 1987 novel *Hot Flashes*, hot flashes incite, are triggered by, and become metaphors for anger, shame, discomfort, guilt, even the atomic bomb. While the protagonist's angst and storyline are distinctly North Ameri-can, the discomfort she expresses in relation to hot flashes is far more global. In this chapter, I apply a biocultural perspective to consider variation in the fre-quency of hot flashes in relation to biological changes associated with aging, as well as culturally influenced factors such as attitudes, stress, breastfeeding pat-terns, smoking habits, and diet.

The Experience

One of the first problems encountered in cross-cultural research on hot flashes is the question of terminology. Vocabulary for symptom experience does not always translate easily across cultures (Davis 1983, 1986; Kaufert and Syrotuik 1981; Melby 2005; Obermeyer, Ghorayeb, and Reynolds 1999). What do women call a hot flash? How do investigators know they are measuring the same phe-nomenon? In the United States, Kronenberg (1990) found that hot flashes were described as sensations of heat, sweating, flushing, anxiety, or chills. Some women also felt irritated, annoyed, or frustrated; some experienced a sense of panic, a feeling of suffocation, or, occasionally, suicidal feelings. Ann Voda tran-scribed the following two interviews in her book *Menopause, Me and You* (1997).

I have different degrees of flashes. Sometimes they are very warm, where I will feel perspiring, but at other times they are just warm and I do not feel perspiring. But I also have an opposite; I also have cold flashes. Sometimes before the hot flash comes I'll have a cold flash, where I get quite cool. So, I dress in layers, so I'm either taking off or I'm putting on. (178)

It is the worst heat. I think I am going to smother. It's a horrible feeling. I feel hot, like a glowing furnace. But the heat is a different kind of heat than you get from running or mowing the lawn; it is very much internal and suffocating. When I have hot flashes, I break out in perspiration—on my feet, legs, in fact everywhere—to the point where sweat runs down my back and down the front. I always carry tissues, towels, handkerchiefs to wipe myself under my eyes, my forehead, anywhere I can wipe. . . . In below-zero weather, I can walk around with my coat open when I have a hot flash but when it is over I'm terribly cold because the sweat starts, and then I'm wet and shivering all over. When people see me this way they think I'm sick, and I'm not. (171)

In Japan, Zeserson (2001) encountered the terms *nobose* or *hoteri,* used by women to describe a generalized flushed feeling, and the expression *kaa to suru* (get hot), which women used in conjunction with qualifiers to describe hot and steamy from the chin up, or suddenly red hot, or the feeling of heat just rising up. There was, however, no precise word for hot flashes, and the words given can be used to describe other forms of overheating. "Nevertheless," Zeserson writes, "when a middle-aged woman who is not bathing, drinking sake, or otherwise ill, fans herself while uttering '*Kak-kak-kak-ka shite iru!* (Whew, I am heating up!),' there is little doubt that she is experiencing some variation of what in English is called *hot flash*" (194).

In Puebla, Mexico, women use the word *bochorno,* which has a root meaning of shame or embarrassment, rather than heat *(calores),* sweat *(sudores),* blushing or suffocating *(sofocos)*—words used to describe hot flashes in other Latin American countries and in Spain. I asked a forty-nine-year-old saleswoman why, in Mexico, women use the word *bochorno.* She replied, "Well, because *calor* [heat] is caused by the environment, whereas a *bochorno* is of the body, *calor de adentro* [inner heat]." Another woman described a hot flash as similar to the inner rush of emotion that occurs when a person is caught in an awkward or embarrassing situation.

Like Zeserson, the research team in Puebla questioned whether Mexican women were describing hot flashes or the generic feeling of being hot. After a week of more careful inquiries, we decided that women were indeed differentiating between ambient heat, kitchen heat, the heat of exercising, and hot flashes when we asked about *bochornos.* For example, a fifty-six-year-old widow described her twelve years of hot flashes in the following way: "When I have a *borchorno,* I feel a lot of heat until I take off my sweater. I sweat a lot. I sweat in my face, chest, back and stomach. At times, when I'm working, I have hot flashes. At home, I have constant small hot flashes." A fifty-year-old secretary explained that she had to cut her hair short because of hot flashes, and she can't wear any makeup. During a hot flash, her face and neck are covered in sweat. She feels that at the moment of a hot flash her blood pressure rises, and this explains why she feels so uncomfortably hot.[1]

According to a sixty-six-year-old mother of seven, "I have hot flashes all of the time, even in the cold, more when I carry out some activity. They started immediately after I stopped menstruating. I have more when I finish my bath. They've always been the same, *muy exagerados,* with a lot of sweat. They start in the front, later behind my head, down to my chest. The heat rises to my head, and I sweat suddenly. They are the same, day and night." A forty-nine-year-old schoolteacher said angrily, "Hot flashes make me feel like I'm on fire, then my husband wants to have relations? No. We sleep in separate beds. I want to be left alone. With the hot flashes, I'm so hot, so hot, then cold. They started with my last menstruation. I wash with cold water two times a day. This has gone on for one year. When menopause begins, no one can understand, not the kids, not the spouse, nobody." Yet descriptions of hot flashes vary widely. One fifty-three-year-old woman stated simply, "I love my hot flashes!" She said she experiences two or three every day. Relatedly, perhaps, she also stated that "going through menopause makes me a little sad—to lose the intensity of hormones" (Leidy Sievert 2001).

Measurement

These descriptions of menopause, from the United States, Japan, and Mexico, demonstrate that hot flashes are a phenomenological event; they are subjectively experienced (Kronenberg 1994). Hot flashes are also physiological events that can be measured apart from women's subjective experiences. Hot flashes are characterized by reddening of the skin and profuse sweating (Whitehead, Whitcroft, and Hillard 1993). They can be measured by changes in palmar (hand) and sternal (chest) skin conductance levels, changes in finger temperature, changes in finger-pulse volume ratios, changes in energy expenditure and respiratory quotient (carbon dioxide production in relation to oxygen consumption), and changes in core body temperature (Carpenter et al. 2004; Casper, Yen, and Wilkes 1979; Freedman 1989; Freedman et al. 1995; Kletzky and Borenstein 1987; Kronenberg 1990; G. W. Molnar 1975; Swartzman, Edelberg, and Kemmann 1990).

During a hot flash, peripheral temperature can increase 4 or 5°C (7 to 9°F) and peripheral vasodilation has been measured in fingers, toes, cheek, forehead, forearm, upper arm, chest, abdomen, back, calf, and thigh (Freedman 2000a).

Elevations in core body temperature right before a hot flash can be measured with a radiotelemetry pill that women swallow (see Freedman 2000a for illustration). The transmitter sends temperature readings to an antenna wrapped around the subject's body as the pill makes its way through the digestive tract (Freedman 1998; Freedman et al. 1995; Freedman and Woodward 1996).

In laboratory settings in Detroit and Amsterdam, the method of objective hot flash measurement that is most highly correlated with the subjective report of a hot flash is sternal skin conductance (de Bakker and Everaerd 1996; Freedman 1989). Sweat rate is recorded from the sternum using a 0.5 V constant voltage circuit and disposable electrodes (Freedman 1989, 2000a). Ambulatory monitoring can also be used to measure changes in skin conductance using electrodes and a small monitor that women carry with them (Carpenter et al. 1999, 2001, 2004; Freedman 1989; Freedman, Woodward, and Norton 1992). In addition to clinical measurements, hot flashes can also be monitored by hot flash diaries (Grisso et al. 1999; Voda 1997:344) and hot flash body diagrams (Voda 1997:346).

In Puebla, Mexico, Robert Freedman helped us set up and carry out sixty-seven studies of hot flashes using sternal skin conductance. We recorded changes in skin conductance level (SCL) on a polygraph. An increase in SCL of two μmho or more in thirty seconds was designated a hot flash. (A μmho is a measure of the electrical conductance of a substance, in this case sweat.) A baseline recording was carried out for thirty minutes, after which two 40 by 60 cm circulating water heating pads were placed on the participant's abdomen and thighs. This was done to provoke hot flashes (Freedman 1989). SCL readings continued for ninety additional minutes. Subjective hot flashes were verbally identified by the participant during the SCL test and *bochorno* was written on the polygraph tracing if they were judged by the participant to be *normal* or *regular* hot flashes (Sievert et al. 2002).

One difference between the experience of hot flashes in Puebla, and the experience of hot flashes in western Massachusetts (Leidy 1997) was the description of how hot flashes began and spread across the body. In western Massachusetts, women described their hot flashes as beginning in their chest and rising upward, or as taking place above their hairline. This matches the description of a "typical" hot flash in the medical literature (as in Elkind-Hirsch 2004). In contrast, women in Puebla described their hot flashes as beginning in their chest and rising upward or, just as often, starting at the back of the neck and coming forward (Sievert et al. 2002). Of the sixty-seven women who participated in the clinical study of hot flashes in Puebla, only thirty-four demonstrated consistent concordance between the subjective reporting of hot flash experience and the objective measurement of hot flashes by sternal skin conductance. The lack of concordance may be explained, in part, by the decision to measure skin conductance on the upper chest (on the basis of studies carried out in Detroit) rather than on the nape of the neck (Sievert et al. 2002).

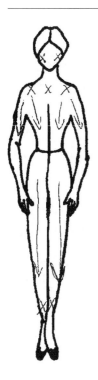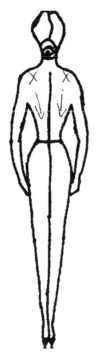

FIGURE 6.1 Body diagram used to map the movement of hot flashes across the body.

During the summer of 2004, I returned to Puebla to monitor hot flashes in thirteen women. During the monitoring session, I asked women to indicate on a body diagram (figure 6.1) how their hot flashes moved across their bodies.[2] Table 6.1 illustrates a sample of the ways in which women described the movement of heat across their bodies. Notice that the first woman (45.9 years) did not describe hot flashes as occurring across her chest. Correspondingly, during the hot flash monitoring, she did not demonstrate a hot flash by sternal skin conductance, but she did demonstrate a hot flash by nuchal (back of neck) skin conductance.

Population Variation

Table 6.2 illustrates variation in hot flash experience and musculo-skeletal-joint pain (see Chapter Five) across fifty-four populations drawn from the literature. This list was first developed for a study of hot flashes in relation to climate (Sievert and Flanagan 2005). Within this sample of studies, frequency of hot flashes varies from 0 percent in Mexico (Beyene 1989) to 82.5 percent in Thailand (Sukwatana et al. 1991). Part of this variation can be explained by the methods used to assess hot flash frequency. For example, some studies reported vasomotor complaints—a combined measure of hot flashes and sweating—rather than hot flashes alone, in the belief that both hot flashes and sweating indicate a disturbance of thermoregulation (Hammar et al. 1984; Kirchengast 1993; Oldenhave et al.

TABLE 6.1

Reports of How Heat Moves across the Body during a Hot Flash, Puebla, Mexico

Age	First Site	Second Site	Third Site	Fourth Site	Fifth Site
45.9	Back of neck	Back of head	Forehead	Hands	
50.7	Front of neck, under breasts, front of thighs	Top of head and back of neck	Upper chest	Middle of back	
50.9	Top of head	Center of chest and back of neck			
51.3	Hands	Upper chest	Forehead	Back of neck	Center of back
54.0	Between breasts	Face	Back of neck	Hands	
54.8	Upper lip	Upper chest	Back of neck	Under breasts	Feet
56.9	Front of neck	Back of neck	Top of head and chest to waist	Hands	
59.75	Back of neck	Back of head and forehead	Chest to waist, arms to elbows		

1993). Although night sweats are physiologically similar to hot flashes, the experience can be very different for women who have to change nightgowns and bed sheets in the middle of the night due to night sweats, but who do not have to change clothes during the day due to hot flashes. A measure of hot flashes and night sweats together may not be equivalent to hot flashes alone. In addition, women have been asked if they were currently experiencing hot flashes ($n = 7$ studies), if they had experienced hot flashes during the past year ($n = 1$), during the past six months ($n = 1$), during the past four weeks ($n = 11$), during the past two weeks ($n = 13$), or if they had ever experienced hot flashes ($n = 21$). One study specified hot flashes "at the time their periods stopped or since periods became irregular" (Staropoli et al. 1998). When it was possible to separate "current" from "ever" hot flash frequency (as in Feldman, Voda, and Gronseth 1985), "current" hot flash frequency was reported in table 6.2. When the time frame was unclear, hot flash frequency was recorded as "ever."

When hot flash frequencies were divided into two categories—within the past month ($n = 31$ studies) and for a longer duration ($n = 23$)—hot flash frequencies

TABLE 6.2

Percentage of Women Reporting Hot Flashes and Somatic Pain

Country (Site)	N	Ages	Study Sample[a]	Time Period Used to Assess Symptom Frequencies	Percentage of Women Reporting Hot Flashes	Percentage of Women Reporting Somatic Pain	Source
Australia (Brisbane)	381	45–54	Repres.	2 weeks prior	25	49 (back pain)	O'Connor et al. (1995)
Australia (Melbourne)	549	45–55	Repres.	2 weeks prior	32	37 (back pain) 49 (joint pain)	Dennerstein et al. (1993)
Austria (Vienna)	142	38–61	Clinical	Current	73.6	58 (muscle pain) 29 (joint pain)	Kirchengast (1993)
Canada (Manitoba)	1,326	45–59	Repres.	2 weeks prior	31	27 (back pain) 31.4 (joint pain)	Avis et al. (1993)
Finland (Helsinki)	1,713	45–65	Repres.	2 weeks prior	28	27 (backache) 27 (joint ache)	Hemminki, Topo, and Kangas et al. (1995)
Ghana (Accra)	123	Meno-pausal	Comm.	Ever	56.5	(Not asked)	Kwawukume, Ghosh, and Wilson (1993)
Greece (Stira, Evia)	66	38–59	Comm.	Ever	72.7	(Not asked)	Beyene (1989)
Hong Kong	427	40–55	Comm.	4 weeks prior	10.2	(Not asked)	Boulet et al. (1994)

(continued)

TABLE 6.2

Percentage of Women Reporting Hot Flashes and Somatic Pain (*continued*)

Country (Site)	N	Ages	Study Sample[a]	Time Period Used to Assess Symptom Frequencies	Percentage of Women Reporting Hot Flashes	Percentage of Women Reporting Somatic Pain	Source
India (Bombay)	495	55 (+/−9)	Comm.	Current	15	(Not asked)	Bharadwaj, Kendurkar, and Vaidya (1983)
Indonesia	346	40–60	Comm.	4 weeks prior	9.8	(Not asked)	Boulet et al. (1994)
Indonesia (Bandung)	1,025	40–55	Comm.	4 weeks prior	10.9	(Not asked)	Agoestina and van Keep (1984)
Indonesia (Java)	297	51.2 (ave.)	Comm.	Ever	17.5	(Not reported)	Flint and Samil (1990)
Indonesia (Sumatra)	306	52.7 (ave.)	Comm.	Ever	24.8	(Not reported)	Flint and Samil (1990)
Japan (Kobe, Kyoto, Nagano)	1,316	45–55	Comm.	2 weeks prior	12.3	24 (back pain) 15 (joint pain)	Lock (1993)
Korea (Seoul)	500	40–60		4 weeks prior	38.5	(Not asked)	Boulet et al. (1994)
Lebanon (Beirut)	271	45–55	Repres.	4 weeks prior	49	44 (joint pain)	Obermeyer, Ghorayeb, and Reynolds (1999)
Malaysia (Kual)	401	40–60	Comm.	4 weeks prior	30	(Not asked)	Boulet et al. (1994)
Mexico (Puebla)	755	40–60	Comm.	2 weeks prior	50	56 (back pain) 56 (joint aches)	Sievert (2001a)

Location	N	Age range	Sample	Recall	%	Symptom	Reference
Mexico (rural Yucatan)	71	33–57	Comm.	Ever	0	(Not asked)	Beyene (1989)
Mexico (Yucatan)	202	35–59	Comm.	Ever	31	55 (back pain)	Canto-de-Cetina, Canto-Cetina, and Polanco-Reyes (1998)
Netherlands (Utrecht)	2,900 / 568	40–44 / 54–69	Repres.	1 year / Current	20.4	(Not asked)	den Tonkelaar, Seidell, and van Noord (1996)
New Zealand (Auckland)	50	48–75	Comm.	Ever	80	50 (aching muscles and joints)	Emmens (1998)
Nigeria (Oyo State)	563	44–87	Comm.	Ever	30	39.6 (joint and bone pains)	Okonofua, Lawal, and Bamgbose (1990)
Norway (Oslo)	1,886	45–55	Repres.	6 months prior	65	55 (muscle and joint pains)	Holte (1991)
Pakistan (Karachi)	650	30–55	Comm.	Ever	36	10 (severe back pain)	Wasti et al. (1993)
Singapore	420	40–60	Comm.	4 weeks prior	14.5	(Not asked)	Boulet et al. (1994)
Slovenia (Selška Valley)	58	32–85	Comm.	2 weeks prior	24	59 (back pain) / 53 (joint aches)	Sievert et al. (2004)
Spain (Alcobendas)	1,248	45–65	Comm.	Ever	47.5	(Not reported)	Barroso Benítez (2003)
Spain (Madrid)	1,500	45–55	Comm.	Ever	71	(Not reported)	Martín (1996) cited in Barroso Benítez (2003)

(continued)

TABLE 6.2

Percentage of Women Reporting Hot Flashes and Somatic Pain *(continued)*

Country (Site)	N	Ages	Study Sample[a]	Time Period Used to Assess Symptom Frequencies	Percentage of Women Reporting Hot Flashes	Percentage of Women Reporting Somatic Pain	Source
Sweden (Linköping)	1,469	60–62	Repres.	Current	27	(Not asked)	Berg et al. (1988)
Sweden (Linköping)	1,118	52–54	Repres.	Current	57	(Not asked)	Hammar et al. (1984)
Sweden (Göteborg)	1,413	40–66	Repres.	Ever	38.9	(Not asked)	Hagstad and Janson (1986)
Taiwan	398	40–60		4 weeks prior	21.4	(Not asked)	Boulet et al. (1994)
Tanzania (Muhez)	50	45–62	Comm.	Ever	82	80 (backache) 72 (joint pain)	Moore and Kombe (1991)
Thailand (Bangkok)	248	40–59	Comm.	2 weeks prior	26.6	53 (back pain) 55 (joint pain)	Punyahotra, Dennerstein, and Lehert (1997)
Thailand (Bangkok)	119	59 (+/−7)	Comm.	Ever	37.7	(Not asked)	Chaikittisilpa et al. (1997)
Thailand (Bangkok)	614	40+	Comm.	Ever	82.5	48 (numbness of extremities)	Sukwatana et al. (1991)
The Philippines (Manila)	500	40–60	Comm.	4 weeks prior	30.2	(Not asked)	Boulet et al. (1994)

Location	N	Age	Sample	Time frame	%	Symptom	Reference
Turkey (Ankara)	1,500	41–70	Clinical	Ever	73.9	82 (muscle-joint-bone pain)	Carda et al. (1998)
UK (Aberdeen)	221	40–60	Clinical	Current	24.4	33 (backache) (joint pain)	Thompson, Hart, and Durno 25 (1973)
United Arab Emirates	742	40+	Comm.	Ever	45.1	22 (joint pain)	Rizk et al. (1998)
U.S. (Chicago)	153	35–69	Comm.	2 weeks prior	41	52 (backaches) 69 (joint aches)	Wilbur et al. (1998)
U.S. Japanese (Hawaii)	346	35–60	Repres.	Current	16	12 (history of arthritis)	Goodman, Stewart, and Gilbert (1977)
U.S. White (Hawaii)	332	35–60	Repres.	Current	22	21 (history of arthritis)	Goodman Stewart, and Gilbert (1977)
U.S. Japanese (Los Angeles)	811	40–55	Repres.	2 weeks prior	11.8	50 (stiffness)	Avis et al. (2001) Gold et al. (2000)
U.S. (Mass.)	8,050	45–55	Repres.	2 weeks prior	34.8	30 (back pain) 39 (joint pain)	Avis et al. (1993)
U.S. Hispanic (NJ)	1,859	40–55	Repres.	2 weeks prior	26	48 (stiffness)	Avis et al. (2001) Gold et al. (2000)
U.S. (NC)	334	41–75	Repres.	Ever	71	(Not asked)	Schwingl, Hulka, and Harlow (1994)
U.S. Chinese (Oakland)	625	40–55	Repres.	2 weeks prior	15.5	48 (stiffness)	Avis et al. (2001) Gold et al. (2000)

(continued)

TABLE 6.2 (continued)
Percentage of Women Reporting Hot Flashes and Somatic Pain (continued)

Country (Site)	N	Ages	Study Sample[a]	Time Period Used to Assess Symptom Frequencies	Percentage of Women Reporting Hot Flashes	Percentage of Women Reporting Somatic Pain	Source
U.S. (RI)	233	45–65	Comm.	Ever	67	(Not asked)	Staropoli et al. (1998)
U.S. (San Diego, CA)	589	50–89	Repres.	Ever	73.9	(Not asked)	von Mühlen, Kritz-Silverstein, and Barrett-Conner (1995)
U.S. African Am. (Philadelphia)	218	35–48	Repres.	4 weeks prior	38	(Not reported)	Grisso et al. (1999)
U.S. White (Philadelphia)	218	35–48	Repres.	4 weeks prior	24	(Not reported)	Grisso et al. (1999)
U.S. (Minneapolis)	594	35–60	Repres.	Current	62	(Not reported)	Feldman, Voda, and Gronseth (1985)

[a]Samples are Repres(entative), Comm(unity/convenience), or Clinical.

were lower in populations where questionnaires limited hot flash experience to less than a month before interview. Among women who reported hot flashes during the last two to four weeks before interview, 28.1 percent reported hot flashes (n = 31 studies) compared with 52.7 percent of women who reported hot flash frequencies during the last six months or longer (n = 23, $p < .01$) (Sievert and Flanagan 2005).

In several instances, we had to add together severe, moderate, and mild hot flash frequencies to attain one number (see Chaikittisilpa et al. 1997). At times, we computed hot flash frequency from subgroup reports (Agoestina and van Keep 1984; Dennerstein et al. 1993; Feldman, Voda, and Gronseth 1985; Goodman, Stewart, and Gilbert 1977; Hagstad and Janson 1986; Hammar et al. 1984; Moore and Kombe 1991; Wasti et al. 1993). As the age ranges suggest, some samples include premenopausal, perimenopausal, and postmenopausal women. Other studies were limited to postmenopausal participants (such as Okonofua, Lawal, and Bamgbose 1990; Schwingl, Hulka, and Harlow 1994). An additional caveat is that some samples include women who were taking hormone therapy and other samples do not. Use of HT can diminish hot flash experience, resulting in lowered frequencies (O'Connor et al. 1995), although this is not always the case (Sievert 2003).

Some samples are representative of a country or large city (n = 21 studies). Others are community or convenience samples (n = 28) or samples drawn from clinics (n = 3). Sampling strategies included random sampling of telephone numbers (Dennerstein et al. 1993; Feldman, Voda, and Gronseth 1985; Grisso et al. 1999), random sampling from population registers (Hagstad and Janson 1986; Holte 1991; O'Connor et al. 1995), mailing questionnaires to entire communities (Berg et al. 1988), and sampling from clinical records (Rizk et al. 1998), from general practices (Thompson, Hart, and Durno 1973), from a menopause center (Carda et al. 1998), and from outpatient waiting areas (Moore and Kombe 1991; Punyahotra, Dennerstein, and Lehert 1997; Staropoli et al. 1998). In Puebla, Mexico, we recruited women from public parks, markets, and streets (Sievert and Hautaniemi 2003). In Slovenia we went to the house of every eligible woman in four mountain villages and spoke with 80 percent of the women who were aged thirty-five years or older. A small number of women were also recruited from the streets of two villages in the valley below (Sievert et al. 2004).

It is of interest that the frequency of reported hot flashes did not significantly vary by sampling strategy, although the three clinical samples appear to have a higher reported hot flash frequency (57.3 percent) compared with the representative and community/convenience studies combined (37.8 percent) (Sievert and Flanagan 2005). It has generally been believed that samples drawn from clinical settings result in higher symptom frequencies (S.E. Ballinger 1985); however, this is not always the case. In western Massachusetts, for example, we carried out a pilot study to compare symptom frequencies between opportunistic samples of women aged forty to sixty years drawn from a doctor's office, other health care delivery sites, and the general community (Leidy, Canali, and Callahan 2000). Women in the sample drawn from the doctor's office were less educated, twice as likely to smoke, twice as likely to be using HT, and three times as likely to have had a hysterectomy compared with the sample drawn from schools and community groups. In open-ended interviews, however, women recruited from the doctor's office were not more likely to report *ever* having experienced hot flashes, sweating episodes, or mood changes in association with menopause compared with the other samples. Similarly, when women were asked to think back over the past two weeks, there were no significant differences among the samples for recall of hot flashes, cold sweats, trouble sleeping, vaginal dryness, or feeling depressed.

We learned that 78 percent of the women recruited from school districts and community groups spoke with a doctor about menopause. In other words, had we been recruiting at the time of their visit to the physician, they could have been recruited from a doctor's office rather than from their workplace. We concluded that, as a result of pervasive pharmaceutical advertising and health education during the time the study took place, women in western Massachusetts were hearing about the benefits of HT and speaking to their physician about menopause—whether or not they were experiencing symptoms that they associated with menopause (Leidy, Canali, and Callahan 2000). It would be interesting to know if this is still the case now that risks of HT are more widely understood. The implication of that study, carried out in the 1990s, is that, in some populations, "clinical" samples will not demonstrate higher symptom frequencies. However, this conclusion is culture-specific and depends on the pervasiveness and content of "education" women receive regarding menopause as a risk factor for osteoporosis and other chronic conditions.

A fair amount of the variation in hot flash frequency across populations can be explained by differences in methodology. Nevertheless, when questions about hot flashes are asked in the same way, variation in hot flash frequencies remains, both between and within populations. The biocultural approach is the best way to examine symptom variation. Figure 6.2 shows the model that I have been using to understand hot flash experience in Puebla, Mexico.

The Biology

Hot flashes do not just happen at menopause. Hot flashes can occur abruptly whenever estrogen levels fall—for example, after the removal of both ovaries (Kronenberg 1990). According to Naftolin, Whitten, and Keefe (1994), following childbirth, the mother's sex steroids rapidly decline, and women experience vaginal dryness, hot flashes, and sleep disturbances. Premenopausal women in their twenties and thirties sometimes complain of hot flashes during the luteal

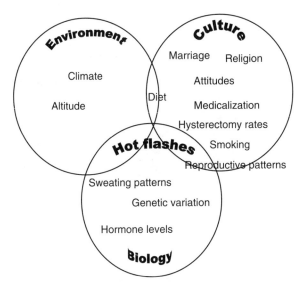

FIGURE 6.2 Biocultural model of how the environment, culture, and biology interact to influence the expression of hot flashes.

phase (when estrogen withdrawal occurs just before menstruation; see figure 2.2), even though their menstrual cycles are regular (Casper, Graves, and Reid 1987; Freeman et al. 2001; Guthrie et al. 1996; Hahn, Wong, and Reid 1998; Kronenberg 1990). Hot flashes also can be experienced by men after orchidectomy (removal of testes) or the administration of a gonadotrophic releasing hormone agonist (Ginsburg and O'Reilly 1983; Linde et al. 1981). An agonist is a drug that can mimic the action of a naturally occurring substance by binding to a cell receptor and triggering a response by the cell. Finally, a self-administered questionnaire mailed to women aged forty-five to fifty found that tubal sterilization ("getting your tubes tied") was associated with hot flashes (Wyshak 2004). Most epidemiologic studies have not found menstrual abnormalities following tubal sterilization procedures (Gentile, Kaufman, and Helbig 1998; Peterson et al. 2000). Some evidence indicates, however, that some sterilization surgeries result in a disruption of blood flow and nerve supply to the ovary (Huggins and Sondheimer 1984). These complications may result in lowered estrogen production by the ovaries (Cattanach 1985) which can result in menopause-like symptoms.

As described in Chapter Two, with advancing age follicular estrogen levels decline and FSH levels rise (Korenman, Sherman, and Korenman 1978; Longcope et al. 1986; Rannevik et al. 1995). Hot flashes are associated with declining estrogen levels (Whitehead, Whitcroft, and Hillard 1993) and rising FSH levels (Guthrie et al. 1996). However, not all women with low estrogen levels and high FSH levels experience hot flashes (Freedman 2000a), and women complaining of hot flashes cannot always be differentiated from asymptomatic women on the basis

TABLE 6.3

Frequency of Hot Flashes in Percent by Country and Menopause Status (with Definitions of Menopause Status Given for Each Study)

Country	Premenopausal	Perimenopausal	Postmenopausal
Australia[a] (Dennerstein et al. 1993)	9.8 (n = 316) Unchanged menstrual flow and frequency, 12 months	31.5 (n = 549) Changes in menstrual frequency and/or flow in past 12 months	39.4 (n = 355) No menses in prior 12 months
Australia[b] (Guthrie et al. 1996)	13 (n = 53) Unchanged menstrual flow and frequency, 12 months	37 (n = 224) Change in menstrual frequency and/or flow in past 12 months	62 (n = 68) No menses in prior 12 months
Lebanon (Obermeyer, Ghorayeb, and Reynolds 1999)	37 (n = 137) Menses in 2 months prior to survey	42 (n = 27) Menses in the 3–11 months prior to survey and irregular	60 (n = 101) No menses in prior 12 months
Sweden (Hagstad and Janson 1986)	18 (n = 640) Menses in 2 months prior to survey	59 (n = 58) Menses in 3–5 months prior to survey	60 (n = 490) No menses in prior 6 months
Thailand (Punyahotra, Dennerstein, and Lehert 1997)	17 (n = 127) Menses with usual regularity during past year	55 (n = 22) Menstrual cycles changed in frequency during past year	33 (n = 99) No menses in prior 12 months
United States SWAN (Gold et al. 2000)	19.4 (n = 4,497) Menses in past 3 months, no irregularity	36.9 (n = 3,547) Menses in past 3 months, irregular 56.8 (n = 611) Menses in past 4 to 12 months	48.8 (n = 1,753) No menses in prior 12 months

[a]Cross-sectional results, Melbourne Women's Midlife Health Project.
[b]Longitudinal results, Melbourne Women's Midlife Health Project.

of hormone profiles (Ballinger, Browning, and Smith 1987). Hot flashes are also experienced in relation to pulses of pituitary LH (although these are not causal), increased levels of brain norepinephrine, and possibly changes in plasma beta-endorphin levels (Casper, Graves, and Reid 1987; Erlik, Meldrum, and Judd 1982; Freedman 1998, 2000a; Kronenberg 1994; Tepper et al. 1992).

In general, women who are in the midst of the menopausal transition (Avis, Crawford, and McKinlay 1997; O'Connor et al. 1995) or who are postmenopausal (Hammar et al. 1984) experience more hot flashes than do women who are premenopausal, as illustrated in table 6.3. In Puebla, Mexico, 38 percent of premenopausal women reported hot flashes during the two weeks before interview compared with 57 percent of naturally postmenopausal and 59 percent of surgically postmenopausal women ($p < 01$).

The putative physiological trigger for hot flashes is a core body temperature elevation acting within a reduced thermoneutral zone—the temperature range in which a woman neither shivers nor sweats (Freedman 2000a,b; Freedman and Blacker 2002). Freedman and Krell (1999) measured this thermoneutral zone in two sessions using a temperature-controlled room where the temperature started at 23°C (73.4°F) and rose to 26°C (78.8°F), then started at 23°C and fell to 4°C (39.2°F). The sweating threshold was defined as the first measurable detection of sweating using a capacitive humidity sensor over the sternum; shivering was measured by electromyographic signals; core body temperature was measured by a rectal thermister probe and a radiotelemetry pill. Twelve postmenopausal women with hot flashes demonstrated a significantly lower sweating threshold—in other words, they sweat more easily as the temperature in the room increased—compared with eight postmenopausal women without hot flashes. The women with hot flashes demonstrated an average interthreshold zone in core body temperature (between sweating and shivering) of 0°C, while women without hot flashes demonstrated an average thermoneutral zone in core body temperature of 0.4°C. The authors suggest that the mechanism behind this difference is brain norepinephrine, which has been shown to narrow the width of the thermoneutral zone in animal studies (Freedman and Krell 1999). Both clonidine (a blood pressure medication also used to manage hot flashes) and estrogen raise the core body temperature sweating threshold in symptomatic women and therefore alleviate hot flashes (Freedman and Blacker 2002; Freedman and Dinsay 2000). Figure 6.3 illustrates the change in thermoneutral zone that is thought to trigger hot flashes.

Correlates of Hot Flashes

As noted in Chapter Three, variables associated with hot flashes in one study may not be associated with hot flashes in another study, because the variables of interest may take on different significance within the contexts of particular

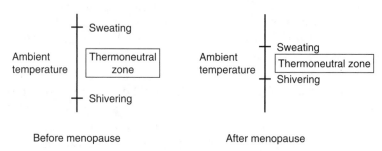

FIGURE 6.3 The body's core temperature thermoneutral zone. Women with a narrowed thermoneutral zone sweat more easily and are more likely to experience hot flashes during the menopause transition.

cultures or age cohorts. That said, progress has nevertheless been made in understanding how some variables are associated with the experience of hot flashes during the menopause transition. Explanations for cross-cultural variation in the frequency of hot flashes have included history of premenstrual symptoms (discussed in Chapter One), climate (Agoestina and van Keep 1984; Boulet et al. 1994; Martin et al. 1993; Oldenhave and Jaszmann 1991; Rizk et al. 1998; Sievert and Flanagan 2005), smoking habits (Dennerstein et al. 1993), socioeconomic status and level of education (Avis, Crawford, and McKinlay 1997; Dennerstein et al. 1993; Schwingl, Hulka, and Harlow 1994; Wilbur et al. 1998), breastfeeding patterns (Lancaster and King 1992), the amount and type of phytoestrogens in the diet (Knight, Lyons Wall, and Eden 1996; Nagata et al. 1999), attitudes toward menstruation, menopause, and aging (Lock 1993), and the medicalization of menopause (Obermeyer 2000).

Maintaining a biocultural perspective and a lifespan approach while examining the frequency of a complaint measured at a particular point in time allows us to more fully understand the data gathered. If hot flashes are measured in July, are these reflective of a general relationship between hot flashes and latitude (mean annual temperature or seasonality)? Do hot flashes reflect smoking habits at the time of menopause, or are there residual effects of early smoking on the endocrine system? Do women have to ingest high levels of phytoestrogen for all of their lives to adequately absorb the phytoestrogenic compounds into their systems? Does body mass index at puberty affect estrogen levels, and do population-specific levels of estrogen affect later hot flash frequencies? At what point do attitudes form that affect the experience of menopause later in the lifespan? As seen in Chapter Four, it is not necessarily at the moment of menopause that variables have the most influence. Biology can be shifted, influenced, and molded at any point in the lifespan, including the prenatal period (Cameron and Demerath 2002; Worthman and Kuzara 2005).

Climate

Previous studies have shown that menopausal hot flashes are more frequent in warm ambient temperatures (Kronenberg and Barnard 1992; G. W. Molnar 1981), and hot flashes can be provoked by body heating (Freedman 1989). If, as Robert Freedman's work in the laboratory suggests, hot flashes are triggered by small elevations of core body temperature within a narrowed thermoneutral zone (Freedman and Blacker 2002; Freedman and Krell 1999), then it follows that as a result of physiological acclimatization, women in different climates may develop different thermoneutral zones or a different degree of sensitivity to temperature change that ultimately affects population-level measures of hot flash frequency.

As mentioned, table 6.2 was first compiled for a test of hot flash frequencies in relation to the average temperature of the hottest month (the monthly mean of the daily temperature in the hottest month of the year), the average temperature of the coldest month (the monthly mean of the daily temperature in the coldest month of the year), the difference between the hottest and coldest months, and the average annual temperature (the yearly mean of the daily temperature) (Sievert and Flanagan 2005). Using simple linear regression equations, and limiting studies to only those with participants aged sixty or younger, we were able to show that average temperature of the coldest month was a significant predictor of hot flash frequency ($p < .01$), explaining 29.2 percent of the variation in hot flash frequency. Women living in colder climates reported more hot flashes (Sievert and Flanagan 2005).

When regressions were carried out using all studies but controlling for the method of hot flash assessment used (within the past two or four weeks versus over a longer duration), average temperature of the coldest month remained a significant predictor ($p < .01$) explaining part of the variation in hot flash frequencies (figure 6.4). Difference in temperature between the hottest and coldest months (seasonality) and mean annual temperature were also significant predictors. Women living in seasonal climates reported more hot flashes. These results suggest that acclimatization to temperature explains part of the population variation in hot flash frequency. Following Freedman's hypothesis, the findings imply that the thermoneutral zone (between shivering and sweating) does not narrow to quite the same degree among menopausal women living in warmer climates, or that women in seasonal climates are more sensitive to temperature change, compared with menopausal women living in colder or less seasonal climates.

In gathering data for figure 6.4 we were unable to control for BMI and occupation (for example, working indoors versus working outdoors), because most investigators do not publish those variables. Thus the role of fat as an insulator and the role of cultural buffers such as air conditioning and central heating could not be addressed. In addition, if developmental acclimatization (adaptation to the environment) is responsible for physiological changes affecting hot flash frequencies, then hot flash frequencies would reflect country (or latitude)

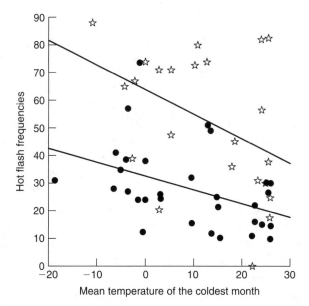

FIGURE 6.4 Variation in hot flash frequency in relation to temperature of the cold-est month (Sievert and Flanagan 2005). Circles represent studies where women were asked about hot flashes during the two or four weeks before interview. Stars represent studies where women were asked about hot flashes during the six months or year before interview, or "ever."

of origin rather than country (or latitude) of residence, a hypothesis difficult to test with the data available. Clothing customs may also affect degree of acclima-tization. A final concern is that the season in which the data were collected was not always published. If acclimatization effects are short term, they may not be adequately examined without controlling for the season of data collection. Nev-ertheless, it appears that the mean daily temperature of the coldest month of the year explains about 29 percent of the variation in hot flash frequency, per-haps due to the process of acclimatization.

Ethnicity

Few studies have compared variation in hot flash frequency between women of different ethnicities living in the same location. Flint and Garcia (1979) showed that middle-class Cuban American women in New Jersey reported more symp-toms in relation to menopause than did middle-class Jewish American women living in the same state. On the other hand, Madeleine Goodman (1980) did not find a difference in symptoms reported by Japanese American and white American women living in Hawaii. More African American than white women reported hot flashes in Philadelphia (38 percent versus 25 percent, $p = 0.01$), but ethnicity did not predict variation in hot flash frequency after controlling for FSH levels, anxiety, alcohol use, BMI, and parity (Freeman et al. 2001). In the multisite SWAN study, African Americans recruited from Pittsburgh, Boston, Detroit, and Chicago reported more hot flashes/night sweats (45.6 percent, n = 3,650) compared with Hispanic women recruited from New Jersey (35.4 percent, n = 1,712), Chinese women from Oakland (20.5 percent, n = 542), Japanese women from Los Angeles (17.6 percent, n = 707), or white women from all seven sites (31.2 percent, n = 3,650) (Gold et al. 2000). In logistic regression analyses, controlling for age, education, health, and ability to pay for basics, African American women were significantly more likely to report a vasomotor symptom than white women, and women of Japanese and Chinese ethnicity were significantly less likely to report a vasomotor symptom than white women measured at the same site. Hispanic women did not differ significantly from non-Hispanic white women at the same site (Avis et al. 2001).

Smoking Habits, Coffee, and Alcohol Intake

A number of studies have noted a link between smoking and hot flashes (Avis, Crawford, and McKinlay 1997; Dennerstein et al. 1993; Freeman et al. 2001; Schwingl, Hulka, and Harlow 1994; Sievert et al. 2002; Staropoli et al. 1998), so that women who smoke are more likely to report hot flashes. These responses could be due to the antiestrogenic effect of smoking (Baron and Greenberg 1987; McMahon et al. 1982). On the other hand, not all studies have noted a link between hot flashes and smoking (Guthrie et al. 1996).

Caffeine has been characterized as a trigger for hot flashes in some studies (Sievert and Hautaniemi 2003); however, Guthrie et al. (1996) found that women experiencing hot flashes several times a day had a lower mean intake of caffeine compared with women who had experienced no hot flashes in the past two weeks. In our clinical study of hot flashes by sternal skin conductance in Puebla, Mexico, we found that smoking and coffee intake were highly correlated. When both smoking and coffee consumption were entered into regression models, coffee was selected as the significant predictor of subjective hot flashes. Note that coffee was a significant predictor of subjective, not objective, hot flash experience. We concluded that coffee intake and associated smoking habits may affect the perception of hot flashes in a way that is dissociated from the objective measurement of sweating by sternal skin conductance (Sievert et al. 2002). In other words, coffee intake was significantly associated with *the perception* of hot flashes, whereas coffee intake was not associated with the objective demonstration of a hot flash by sternal skin conductance. Women who drink coffee may feel more hot flashes.

Alcohol intake has also been associated with higher hot flash frequencies in some (Freeman et al. 2001; Schwingl, Hulka, and Harlow 1994; Sievert et al. 2006) but not all (Guthrie et al. 1996) studies. There is general consensus that alcohol raises estrogen levels (Gill 2000); therefore one might expect *fewer* hot flashes with moderate alcohol consumption.

Socioeconomic Status and Education Level

From a biocultural perspective, the relationship between education or socio-economic status and hot flash frequency is more difficult to explain than, for example, the relationship between smoking habits and hot flash experience. However, women with less education are significantly more likely to experience hot flashes at menopause (Avis, Crawford, and McKinlay 1997; Dennerstein et al. 1993; Gold et al. 2000; Schwingl, Hulka, and Harlow 1994; Wilbur et al. 1998). For example, in a study of hot flashes among African American and white women in Philadelphia, 51 percent of women with less than a high school education reported hot flashes, compared with 29 percent of women with a high school education or more (Freeman et al. 2001). Both ethnicity and education were significant risk factors for hot flashes in multivariate logistic regression models (Grisso et al. 1999).

Consistent with these findings, women with fewer years of education in Puebla ($n = 755$) were significantly more likely to report hot flashes and cold sweats. However, in the clinical study of hot flashes among a subset of women ($n = 67$), women with *more* years of education were more likely to demonstrate hot flashes via sternal skin conductance.

Prolonged Lactation

It has been hypothesized, on the basis of cross-cultural observations, that hormonal fluctuations of the perimenopause are masked by circulating levels of prolactin and oxytocin when women breastfeed their last infant into the perimenopausal period (Lancaster and King 1992; Lancaster and Lancaster 1983). It has been difficult, however, to test this hypothesis within a population. In the clinical test of hot flashes carried out in Puebla ($n = 67$) there was a relationship between subjective hot flash experience and duration of breastfeeding the last child—women who breastfed for a shorter period of time were more likely to report hot flashes (Sievert et al. 2002).

However, this relationship was not demonstrated among the 755 women interviewed in the community sample. One reason for this was the high rate of tubal ligations within this population (42.5 percent), carried out at an average age of thirty-three years. Hence, only 19 percent of the sample had given birth after the age of thirty-five. Women with a last birth at thirty-five years or later, who breastfed their last child for twelve months or longer, were just as likely to report hot flashes (53 percent, 26/49) during the two weeks prior to interview as were women who had given birth to their last child prior to age thirty-five or who had not breastfed for an entire year (51 percent, 302/590) (Sievert 2003).

Diet

Diet has been a particularly confusing area of study in relation to hot flashes. The interest in diet and hot flashes increased dramatically after Margaret Lock's report that women in Japan had fewer and less severe menopausal symptoms than woman in the United States and Canada (Lock 1993). It was suggested by many investigators that Japanese women had fewer hot flashes because of the high amount of soy they were eating. Soy is rich in phytoestrogens (plant estrogens). Phytoestrogens have chemical structures that are very similar to estrogens produced by the body, and they exert similar, but weaker, chemical effects. The three classes of phytoestrogens are coumestans (sprouts), lignands (whole grains, fruits, vegetables, flaxseed), and isoflavones (soy beans and legumes) (Adlercreutz et al. 1992; Knight, Lyons Wall, and Eden 1996). The consumption of phytoestrogens influences estrogen metabolism (demonstrated in metabolite excretion) and serum hormone concentrations (Brooks et al. 2004). Because Japanese women have higher levels of estrogen excretion, it was thought that if women in the United States ate soy, they would have fewer hot flashes; however, short-term studies of soy-product versus placebo consumption and hot flashes have been disappointing (Lu, Tice, and Bellino 2001).

In Puebla, we asked women how many times during the past two weeks they had eaten any of a list of foods. The list included commonly eaten foods that are high in phytoestrogens. For example, during the two weeks before interview, 86 percent of the women ate beans across an average of nine days; 51 percent drank *atole,* a drink made from corn, wheat, or rice, an average of six days; 32 percent ate garbanzo beans an average of one day; and 21 percent ate some sort of soy product an average of four days. In contrast to our expectations, beans, garbanzos, and soy were not associated with hot flash frequency, but women who drank *atole* were significantly less likely to report hot flashes compared with women who did not drink *atole.* When I returned to Mexico, I asked Mexican friends and colleagues why this might be so. *Atole* has phytoestrogens, but compared with soy beans or flaxseed the phytoestrogen content of *atole* is very low. A number of women gave me the same explanation. They said that *atole* warms the body, so women don't notice their hot flashes. These remarks deserve further investigation.

Body Mass Index

As early as the sixth century in Byzantium, variations in age at menopause were noted in accord with body weight (Amundsen and Diers 1973). Contemporary researchers suggest two hypotheses to explain the dual, opposite associations observed between BMI and hot flashes. One hypothesis is endocrinological (hormonal). Heavier women tend to have higher concentrations of estrogens and leaner women tend to have lower concentrations of estrogens because androstenedione (an androgen) is converted to estrone (a weak estrogen) by adipose tissue. In addition, Sylvia Kirchengast and colleagues Hartmann and Huber (1996) found that the sex hormone binding globulin (SHBG) is negatively correlated with body fat in premenopausal women. If heavier women have less SHBG, that means that more sex hormone is unbound, or free, in the body's circulation. In other words, heavier women may have more biologically active, unbound estrogen. Relatedly, women with high levels of obesity have lower levels of FSH (Huerta et al. 1997; Velasco et al. 1990), and in postmenopausal women, LH and FSH correlate negatively with body fat. Kirchengast and colleagues (1996) explain this negative correlation with the observation that heavier women produce more estrogen in their body tissues and, therefore, have lower gonadotropin levels, because there is more negative feedback on LH and FSH secretion. The higher concentrations of estrone in heavier women are thought to diminish hot flashes. Support for this hypothesis is seen in studies where leaner women have been found to have more hot flashes (Campagnoli et al. 1981; Erlik, Meldrum, and Judd 1982; Guthrie et al. 1996; Huerta et al. 1995; Schwingl, Hulka, and Harlow 1994).

The alternative hypothesis could be called biophysical: women who experience hot flashes have a narrower thermoneutral zone—the zone between sweating and shivering as shown in figure 6.3—compared with women who do not experience hot flashes (Freedman 2002; Freedman and Krell 1999). This hypothesis posits that heavier women have more insulation, therefore a narrower thermoneutral zone, and consequently more hot flashes. This hypothesis is supported by many studies in which heavier women have a higher frequency of hot flashes (Carpenter et al. 1998; Chiechi et al. 1997; den Tonkelaar, Seidell, and van Noord 1996; Freeman et al. 2001; Sternfeld, Quesenberry, and Husson 1999; Wilbur et al. 1998). In other studies there is no association between BMI and hot flash frequencies (Grisso et al. 1999; Staropoli et al. 1998), or the association is not present in late perimenopausal or postmenopausal women (Gold et al. 2000).

In Puebla, women with hot flashes during the two weeks before interview were, on average, heavier ($29.2 \, kg/m^2$, s.d. 4.5) than women without hot flashes ($28.6 \, kg/m^2$, s.d. 4.6), although the difference was not significant ($p = 0.07$). Women in the top half ($>28.6 \, kg/m^2$) of the BMI distribution were significantly more likely to report hot flashes (53.8 percent) during the two weeks prior to interview compared with women in the lower half of the BMI distribution (46.5 percent, $p < 0.05$). Heavier women were also more likely to report episodes of cold sweats (34.6 percent versus 26.6 percent, $p < .05$). These findings support the insulation hypothesis, that hot flashes are associated with a greater amount of body insulation and perhaps a narrowed thermoneutral zone.

At present, one can only conclude that the relationship between BMI and hot flashes is still unclear. Different populations demonstrate different associations (positive, negative, and none).

Stressful Life Events

After a broad review, M. S. Hunter (1993:43) concluded that among the most relevant factors influencing a woman's experience at menopause are her social situation and her experience of stressful life events. In Peru, satisfaction with principal life roles was the most important factor associated with attitudes toward menopause (Barnett 1988). In León, Guanajuato, Mexico, perimenopausal women from middle to low socioeconomic levels identified attitudes toward sexuality and family function as the most important factors associated with anxiety (breathlessness, palpitation, tremor, agitation) for menopausal women (Huerta et al. 1995). Other studies have demonstrated the effect of marital (dis)satisfaction on health (Finkler 1994; Kerns et al. 1990), and extensive interviews in Puebla also point to the importance of marriage and family in determining a woman's general well-being and attention to the symptoms of menopause. As Hilma Granqvist noted in 1931, "above all" marriage "is so important and works so much change in the conditions" of women's lives (Granqvist 1931:22).

During the summer of 2004, while monitoring hot flashes in Puebla, a number of my conversations with women drifted to the topic of men. Husbands, these women complained, become "andropáusicos" (they have a shortage of male hormones) and don't want to accept this about themselves. For this reason, men look for younger women. In contrast, "la mujer no busca eso" (the woman does not look for that). One fifty-year-old married woman explained to me that menopause is definitely more difficult if a woman has problems with her husband. She has more anxiety, loneliness, and lower self-esteem. A fifty-four-year-old woman confided that her husband is leaving the house more often. It is extremely upsetting to her, but what can she do? With age, a man gains value. With age, a woman loses value, and her self-esteem falls. When I asked my standard question during the interview, "What symptoms do you have in relation to the end of menstruation?" she answered "I feel less valued—I feel this strongly." She also complained of hot flashes.

Socioeconomic difficulties are also associated with increased symptom frequencies at menopause in a number of studies (Avis, Crawford, and McKinlay 1997; Kuh, Wadsworth, and Hardy 1997; Wilbur et al. 1998). For example, in the multisite SWAN study, all symptoms associated with menopause were increased in women who reported difficulty paying for basic amenities, and the prevalence of symptoms increased with greater difficulty in meeting basic needs (Gold et al. 2000). Again, during the summer of 2004, a forty-five-year-old single mother in Puebla who experiences hot flashes that soak her hair and make her whole body hot explained that life is harder for single women because they can't rest. "I can't. I feel bad, I have a headache, I take an aspirin and continue to work. I'm alone with no one to support me. Jobs go to the young people and there are so many young people." This woman was looking forward to the end of her menstruation, because "My head always hurts. I am always sick. But people say that when menstruation stops, that's when you feel better." Other women similarly connected difficulties at menopause to work-related stress. A fifty-year-old mother of three would like to return to secretarial work but, she explained, women older than forty-five cannot find work. She said that the job hunt "makes me feel like an old woman." Finally, a forty-seven-year-old mother of three thinks that there is probably a connection between her colitis, her hot flashes, and stress related to lack of money. Her husband recently left for the United States, but he has been sending little money home.

Stress was also a topic of conversation during pilot interviews in Hilo, Hawaii, but the conversations did not linger on difficulties with men. Women explained to me that stress did not necessarily make their menopause more difficult. Instead, the transition to menopause seemed to intensify the stress that they experienced in other parts of their lives. As one fifty-seven-year-old Chinese American woman explained to me, she practices breathing deeply and calming herself down, now that she is going through menopause, to avoid over-reacting when family problems arise.

Cultural Attitudes

Attitudes are often assessed by administering agreement scales in conjunction with statements about menopause or aging (Avis, Crawford, and McKinlay 1997; Davis 1983; Hemminki, Topo, and Kangas 1995; Neugarten et al. 1963). Table 6.4 provides an abridged statement list developed in Chicago by Bernice L. Neugarten and colleagues. For each statement, respondents are asked to check whether they (1) agree strongly, (2) agree to some extent, (3) disagree somewhat, or (4) disagree strongly (Neugarten et al. 1963). First published in 1963, this symptom list is now forty years old, yet it continues to be widely used in its original or modified form (Avis, Crawford, and McKinlay 1997; Bell 1995; Sommer et al. 1999).

Davis (1986) found that Newfoundland women were unable to answer questions that required choosing between degrees, such as "definitely agree, agree, don't so much agree, and do not agree." I believe that many Mexican women in Puebla would also have this difficulty. Instead, a different type of attitudinal measure was developed and validated by Bowles (1986) as an alternative way to measure attitudes without requiring study participants to agree or disagree with lists of positive and negative statements. Bowles's list of dichotomies uses a seven-point scale to indicate the degree to which women think each adjective relates to feelings a woman may experience during menopause. The lead-in phrase is, "During menopause a woman feels . . ." The twenty adjective scales are listed in table 6.5. This list of dichotomies can also be presented as a forced choice—either/or (Sievert and Espinosa-Hernandez 2003).

Researchers have repeatedly demonstrated that premenopausal women hold more negative attitudes toward menopause than do postmenopausal women (Bowles 1986; Gannon and Ekstrom 1993; Neugarten et al. 1963; Sievert and Espinosa-Hernandez 2003; Sommer et al. 1999; Wagner et al. 1995). Among studies that have directly examined symptom experience in relation to attitudes, it has been shown that premenopausal negative beliefs about menopause predict depressed mood at the time of menopause (Avis and McKinlay 1991; Dennerstein

TABLE 6.4

Attitudes toward Menopause Checklist

Menopause is an unpleasant experience for a woman.

Women should expect some trouble during the menopause.

In truth, just about every woman is depressed about the change of life.

Women generally feel better after the menopause than they have for years.

A woman gets more confidence in herself after the change of life.

After the change of life, a woman feels freer to do things for herself.

Many women think menopause is the best thing that ever happened to them.

Going through the menopause really does not change a woman in any important way.

Women who have trouble with the menopause are usually those who have nothing to do with their time.

Women who have trouble in the menopause are those who are expecting it.

Women worry about losing their minds during the menopause.

A woman is concerned about how her husband will feel toward her after the menopause.

A woman in menopause is apt to do crazy things she herself does not understand.

Menopause is a mysterious thing which most women don't understand.

If the truth were really known, most women would like to have themselves a fling at this time in their lives.

After the menopause a woman is more interested in sex than she was before.

Source: Neugarten et al. (1963).

et al. 2000; M. S. Hunter 1992). With regard to hot flashes, Avis, Crawford, and McKinlay (1997) found that women who agreed with the statement "Many women become depressed or irritable during the menopause" demonstrated a higher hot flash/night sweat frequency. Women who agreed with the statement "Many women with many interests in life hardly notice the menopause" demonstrated lower frequencies of hot flashes/night sweats. Dennerstein et al. (1993) also found a greater frequency of vasomotor symptoms associated with negative attitudes toward aging or menopause.

In Puebla, we investigated "how a woman feels during menopause." Only seven items were chosen from the list in table 6.5 (Bowles 1986) for inclusion in the Puebla survey and the items were presented as dichotomies (for example,

TABLE 6.5
Menopause Attitude Scale

Important–unimportant	Unattractive–attractive
Passive–active	Pessimistic–optimistic
Clean–dirty	Full–empty
Fresh–stale	Pleasant–unpleasant
Dumb–intelligent	Ugly–beautiful
Sharp–dull	Needed–unneeded
Unsure–confident	Useful–useless
Worthless–valuable	Interesting–uninteresting
High–low	Unsuccessful–successful
Strong–weak	Alive–dead

Source: Bowles (1986).

secure or insecure) (Sievert and Espinosa-Hernandez 2003). The majority of respondents said that a menopausal woman feels "insecure" (66 percent) and "unattractive" (53 percent). Reasons for feeling unattractive included weight gain at menopause. Complained one fifty-seven-year-old respondent, "la menopausia engorda una" (menopause makes one fat). A fifty-one-year-old woman explained that she feels unattractive because of her hot flashes and the "sudor feo" (ugly or awful sweat).

On the other hand, the majority of respondents also said that a menopausal woman is "complete" (62 percent), "necessary" (77 percent), and "successful" (75 percent). In Puebla, women are the primary caretakers of children—until those children marry, maybe in their late twenties or early thirties. Middle-aged women are active caretakers of grandchildren; they maintain extended family relationships and care for ill family members. Among women who chose the word "necessary," a fifty-one-year-old respondent added "for my children." A fifty-three-year-old said that she was "indispensable." Significantly more naturally postmenopausal respondents ($n = 254$) described a woman during menopause as "secure" or a "success," compared with women who had menopause by hysterectomy ($n = 163$) or premenopausal women ($n = 303$), $p < .05$. Natural menopause may bring a comforting sense of closure to some reproductive roles.

Descriptions in Puebla of a woman during menopause as "insecure," "unattractive," "empty," "unnecessary," "boring," or "dead" were not associated with a greater frequency of hot flashes. Only respondents who described the menopausal woman as a "failure" were significantly more likely to report hot flashes (Sievert and Espinoso-Hernandez 2003).

Medicalization

One question raised by the literature is whether or not women in all cultures experience hot flashes in the same way (Kronenberg 1990). Perhaps women do not pay attention to their hot flashes, or do not label a particular sensation to be a hot flash, in cultures where menopause is not a medical event. For example, Yewoubdar Beyene (1986, 1989) found no evidence of hot flash experience among the rural Maya of Yucatán, Mexico, despite hormonal changes with age that were very similar to those measured in the United States (Martin et al. 1993). Beyene, an anthropologist, lived in the Maya village of Chichimilá, population 2,300, near the city of Valladolid, for twelve months, asking questions about menarche, menstruation, and menopause. In contrast, Canto-de-Cetina, a Maya gynecologist, interviewed postmenopausal women in two Yucatan villages, twenty-eight kilometers and forty-two kilometers from the city of Mérida, and reported hot flash frequencies of 28 percent and 33 percent. Canto-de-Cetina and her colleagues (1998) carried out their study in response to Beyene's surprising results. Canto-de-Cetina knew from her medical work near Mérida that Maya women did, in fact, report hot flashes in relation to menopause. Did the women interviewed by the gynecologist have more contact with the health care system? Were they more strongly influenced by the medicalization of menopause?

The concept of medicalization refers to the process whereby aspects of everyday life come under medicine's supervision and influence (Zola 1972, 1983). Through medicalization, the labels "healthy" and "ill" are applied to aspects of human experience that had previously been outside of medicine's domain (Verweij 1999). Medicalization extends the boundaries of medicine by defining experiences in medical terms and by "treating" conditions through medical intervention (Conrad 1992), but it is important to point out that medicalization is an interactive process in which patients participate (Conrad 1992; Griffiths 1999; Purdy 2001; Riessman 1983). The medical management of menopause and the use of HT have been common foci of the critiques of medicalization (Backett-Milburn, Parry, and Mauthner 2000; Bell 1987; Griffiths 1999; Kaufert 1988; Kaufert and Gilbert 1986; Kaufert and Lock 1997; Komesaroff, Rothfield, and Daly 1997; Lock 1993; MacPherson 1985; McCrea 1983; Palmlund 1997a; Rueda 1997; Woods and Mitchell 1999; Worcester and Whately 1992).

Female biology, more so than male biology, is aggressively "treated" by medicine (Foster 1995; Riessman 1983), and in the 1990s HT became increasingly common in the United States (Palmlund 1997b; Woods et al. 1997) as well as in parts of Europe (Rozenberg et al. 2000) and Latin America. For example, in 1999, in the city of Puebla, Dra. Julia Moreno Pacheco spoke on the radio once a month, appeared on TV once a month, and gave an educational conference once a month in a downtown hotel. Her goal was to educate the women of Puebla about chronic diseases associated with menopause (and the benefits of HT). In addition, health concerns associated with menopause are featured prominently in Mexican women's magazines.

The medical management of menopause by HT was promoted through the popular media, self-help books, epidemiology, medical journals, advertising, professional medical societies, the medical profession, and the pharmacuetical industry. The result of this promotion of HT was the creation of a mind-set that linked menopause with not only an option but an obligation to prescribe HT. This attitude was only recently challenged.

HT can result in continued menstruation, changed symptom experience, and health concerns among women of menopausal age. During the 1990s, every open-ended interview I carried out in western Massachusetts concluded with the question: "Do you have any particular concerns, or do you anticipate (or have you experienced) any benefits, with menopause?" Although the question was carefully worded to target menopause, many women started their response by saying, "Well, I don't know whether or not to take hormones." The concerns most often voiced included osteoporosis, cardiovascular disease, fear of memory loss, and breast cancer—concerns women have learned to associate with the end of menstruation as the result of the medicalization of menopause.

The treatment of menopause as an aspect of human variation, rather than as a biomedical event, allows for greater theoretical, methodological, and interpretive breadth. However, any biocultural investigation of age and symptoms associated with the cessation of menses, particularly in an urban environment, will be affected by the medicalization of menopause (Sievert 2003).

An Example of Medicalization: The Treatment of Hot Flashes

Many aspects of human variation, such as childhood growth or blood pressure, enter the medical domain at measurement extremes. Menopause differs in that not only are the extremes of variation cause for medical concern, but the entire cessation of reproduction is treated as a disease event. Questions about variation in age and symptom experience at menopause take on immediate clinical significance.

Physicians may prescribe HT for reasons ranging from the prevention of bone loss, to the prevention of cardiovascular disease, to the delay of Alzheimer's disease (Mueller, Jiménez Zerón Sánchez, and Leidy Sievert 2003).[3] However, hot flashes are the primary menopausal complaint for which women seek medical treatment—they want relief from their symptoms (Kronenberg 1990), and hot flashes are one of the primary reasons that physicians give for prescribing HT (Elinson, Cohen, and Elmslie 1999; Hemminki et al. 1993; Mueller, Jiménez Zerón Sánchez, and Leidy Sievert 2003).

From a biocultural perspective, biomedicine is part of the "culture" that interacts with the biology of menopause. One way that medicine interacts with the biology of menopause is of course through the treatment of menopausal symptoms. HT is an effective treatment for hot flashes, night sweats, and vaginal dryness (Kronenberg 1994). However, menopause has a history of medical attention that precedes the discovery of estrogen. During the nineteenth century, for example, the "change of life" was considered to be a "critical period" that determined the future mental and physical health of all women (Currier 1897; Tilt 1882). By the nineteenth century, hot flashes had long been attributed to the menopause transition, or, more correctly, to the climacteric—the transition from the reproductive to the postreproductive phase of life.

Since the discovery of estrogen, menopause has been defined as a deficiency disease, similar to diabetes or hypothyroidism (Bell 1987; McCrea 1983). Synthetic estrogen replacement became widely available in the 1960s, prescribed so that women could remain "feminine forever" (Wilson 1966), in part to improve the life of their husbands (Cooper 1975; McCrea 1983). During the 1970s the use of estrogen declined dramatically, because of an epidemic of endometrial cancer that was caused by women taking unopposed estrogen, that is estrogen alone (Kennedy, Baum, and Forbes 1985). The use of estrogen therapy (ET) in countries such as Finland continues to increase the risk of hysterectomies (Vuorma et al. 1998), as it did in the United States prior to the use of estrogen/progestin combinations.

When the treatment protocol shifted in the United States to the use of estrogen combined with progestin, HT gained popularity in the 1980s. Progestin demonstrated protection against endometrial cancer, and HT was hailed, for a second time, as a rejuvenator (Nachtigall and Heilman 1986). By 1992 all women were urged to consider HT (American College of Physicians 1992) from the perimenopausal period until the effect of estrogens began to wane, sometime after the age of seventy five (Ettinger and Grady 1993). Menopause became a risk factor for osteoporosis (Nuti and Martini 1993; Pouilles, Tremollieres, and Ribot 1993) and cardiovascular disease (Stevenson, Crook, and Godsland 1993) rather than a disease in and of itself (Worcester and Whatley 1992). The strongest arguments for the use of HT came from cost-benefit analyses that demonstrated reduced social costs specific to osteoporosis and cardiovascular disease among women taking the medication (Daly et al. 1994; Mishell 1989; Notelovitz 1989; Utian 1978).

However, all of this changed as a result of two large prospective, randomized, double-blind, placebo-controlled studies, the Heart and Estrogen/Progestin Replacement Study (HERS) (Grady et al. 2002; Hulley et al. 1998) and the Women's Health Initiative (WHI) (Writing Group 2002). The WHI study was stopped in 2002, in part because of the finding that oral estrogen plus oral progestin (Prempro) increased the risk of coronary heart disease and stroke (Manson et al. 2003; Wassertheil-Smoller et al. 2003). Another long-term study in the United Kingdom,

Australia, and New Zealand (WISDOM) was stopped in 2002 because of the WHI results (White 2002). Although the findings of the HERS and WHI study continue to be debated, it is now widely acknowledged that oral estrogen plus oral progestin increases the risk of breast cancer (Writing Group 2002). Researchers and others interested in the debate for and against the widespread use of HT had been aware of this risk since the mid-1990s (Collaborative Group 1997).

Menopause Induced by Chemotherapy

Women who have undergone chemotherapy are particularly predisposed to hot flashes (Carpenter et al. 2002). Chemotherapy and/or radiation therapy used to treat childhood cancers, breast cancer, cancer of the cervix, Hodgkin's disease, or systemic lupus can also result in an early end to reproductive function (Reichman and Green 1994; Sonmezer and Oktay 2004; Stanford et al. 1987). According to Sonmezer and Oktay (2004), 8 percent of female cancer cases occur under the age of forty years, and chemotherapy during the premenopausal years can result in irreversible damage to the granulosa and theca cells of the ovarian follicle as well as to the oocyte (undeveloped egg). Studies of ovarian tissue have documented the extent of follicle loss following the use of chemotherapeutic agents (Familiari et al. 1993).

Damage to the ovaries occurs not only through direct exposure to radiation, such as abdominal or pelvic irradiation, but through scatter radiation even if the ovaries are outside of the radiation field (Sonmezer and Oktay 2004). Radiation causes a dose-related reduction in the ovarian reserve of primordial follicles (Gosden et al. 1997). Older women are most affected by exposure to chemotherapy and radiation, and are most likely to develop complete ovarian failure, probably because they had fewer oocytes to start with (Schilsky et al. 1981). Relatedly, with advancing age, permanent ovarian damage can be caused by smaller doses of the chemotherapeutic agent. Even among younger women, however, ovarian function will not necessarily return to normal after chemotherapy (Schimmer et al. 1998).

Women who have undergone chemotherapy as part of their treatment for breast cancer are particularly prone to hot flashes (Carpenter et al. 2002). In addition to having an increased potential for early ovarian failure, women who have undergone treatment for breast cancer often take tamoxifen. Tamoxifen functions as an estrogen antagonist in the breast cells, decreasing estrogen levels in the breast tissue.[4] This effect is helpful for women who have breast cancer tumors that contain estrogen receptors, because tamoxifen slows the growth or return of breast cancer. But as an estrogen antagonist, tamoxifen can cause severe estrogen-deficiency symptoms, such as hot flashes. In addition, women who have undergone chemotherapy for breast cancer demonstrate disruptions in their daily hormonal rhythms and body temperature (Carpenter et al. 2001).

Hot flashes are one of the most commonly reported symptoms among women who have completed treatment for breast cancer (Carpenter et al. 1998; Stein et al. 2000). Carpenter and colleagues (1998) found that 65 percent of postmenopausal women treated for breast cancer reported hot flashes, and that 59 percent of women with hot flashes rated their hot flashes as "severe." Hot flashes were most severe in women with a higher BMI, in women who were younger at diagnosis, and in women taking tamoxifen. Stein and colleagues (2000) found a 40 percent hot flash rate among postmenopausal women with breast cancer undergoing chemotherapy and radiotherapy treatment. Of those women with hot flashes, 25 percent rated their hot flashes as "severe." Women with chemo- and radiation-induced hot flashes were younger, and the prevalence of hot flashes significantly predicted poorer sleep patterns, more fatigue, and worse physical health.

In a study comparing hot flash experience between breast cancer survivors and women who had never had breast cancer, hot flashes were more frequent, severe, distressing, and of longer duration among breast cancer survivors (Carpenter et al. 2002). Consistent with the discussion above, more breast cancer survivors (79 percent) were postmenopausal (through natural, surgical, or chemical means) compared with the women who had never been treated for breast cancer (57 percent, $p < .01$). Significantly more breast cancer survivors reported daily hot flashes (65 percent) in comparison with healthy women (16 percent) and, on a scale of zero to ten where 0 = not severe and 10 = extremely severe, breast cancer survivors reported a higher overall hot flash severity of 3.8 (s.d. 3.0) compared with the healthy women's score of 1.4 (s.d. 2.6, $p < .01$).

When breast cancer survivors reported doing something to alleviate their hot flashes, they reported fanning themselves (71 percent), removing clothing to cool off (64 percent), moving to a cooler environment (64 percent), and doing nothing (21 percent). They also tried exercise (57 percent), vitamins (56 percent), diet (30 percent), relaxation and other behavioral methods (24 percent), herbs (9 percent), and massage (6 percent) to reduce the severity and frequency of hot flashes. Breast cancer survivors reported their hot flash treatments to be significantly less effective compared with those of healthy women (an effectiveness of 4.7 versus 9.8 on a scale of 0 to 10) (Carpenter et al. 2002).

As more and more women survive cancers, the results of treatment—early menopause and drug-related hot flashes—will be more common. For example, while piloting a menopause survey in Hilo, Hawaii, with Dan Brown and Lynn Morrison in the summer of 2004, I interviewed nineteen women recruited from the university and a local elementary school and found that two (10.5 percent of the sample) had undergone chemotherapy for cancer and were still trying to control the resulting hot flashes. This finding is a useful reminder that each cohort of women has its own health-related history, and studies carried out over the next decade will have many more cancer survivors compared with, for example, studies carried out in the 1970s and 1980s. Symptom experience at menopause can be dramatically altered by chemotherapy and subsequent tamoxifen use. It is critical that contemporary studies of menopause include questions about past experience with chemotherapy or radiation treatments as more and more women survive their cancers.

Putting It All Together

Why do hot flash frequencies vary so dramatically between and within populations? In Puebla, Mexico, we used logistic regression to examine many variables in relation to hot flash frequency. Significant factors ($p < 0.05$) predicting hot flashes during the two weeks prior to interview were postmenopausal status, a BMI of more than 28.59 kg/m^2, less education, abdominal cramps with menstruation, having spoken with a physician about menopause, and having consumed less *atole* during the two weeks before interview.

As this chapter demonstrates, the holism of the biocultural approach means paying attention to a wide range of variables across a number of lifespan trajectories. In Puebla, the significant factors predicting hot flash occurrence included hormone levels (assuming that menopause status is a proxy for estrogen levels), BMI (a proxy for circulating estrogen levels as well as a measure of body insulation), a history of abdominal cramps with menstruation earlier in the lifespan, seeking medical advice (a less than ideal measure of medicalization), and reduced consumption of one culturally specific food. Freeman et al. (2001) used the same sort of logistic regression model to find the predictors of hot flashes among African American and white women in Philadelphia, but came up with a different list of explanatory variables: FSH levels, BMI, anxiety, alcohol use, and number of children.

Because hot flashes are greatly affected by cultural context, every population will produce a different set of explanatory variables, even if researchers use the same methods. Is it acceptable for women to smoke? Do women have educational opportunities beyond eighth or ninth grade? Can older women find jobs? Do women give birth early in their lifespan or late? What are the foods most commonly eaten by women of menopausal age? What are the culturally specific stressors that women must deal with every day? How do they feel about menstruation and aging? What are the cultural messages about a woman's value? Do health care providers treat menopause as a disease state to be managed or as a natural transition in an active and useful life? Some of these variables could be collected in an etic, checklist sense for cross-population comparisons—for example, smoking or age at childbirth—just as climate was compared in relation to hot flash frequency across fifty-six populations.

In lieu of that type of broad comparison, all menopause researchers would benefit from collecting the same variables for comparison *within* populations.

Then we could ask why a variable may be a significant predictor of hot flashes in one population, but not in another, knowing that all of a certain set of variables have been examined. For example, in Puebla, did we examine alcohol consumption in relation to hot flashes? (Not in the logistic model.) In Philadelphia, did they examine abdominal cramps with menstruation in relation to hot flashes at menopause? (Not in the same way. They asked whether or not women experienced severe premenstrual distress, defined as premenstrual symptoms that impaired usual functioning.) I am not suggesting that we need one single standardized questionnaire for use in all cultures, but that we ask for the same general information and collect the height and weight measurements necessary for computing BMIs wherever we go.

CHAPTER SEVEN

Conclusions and Future Directions

Why do human females experience a universal menopause followed by a very long period of postreproductive life? Does nutrition explain variation in age at menopause across populations, or is variation in age at menopause between developed and developing countries wholly an artifact of different research methodologies? Why do some women experience hot flashes while others do not? Some populations have a higher frequency of hot flashes compared with others; is social stress a key part of the explanation? The systematic study of menopause across populations is still a relatively young area of research, but as more investigators collect similar dependent (outcome) and independent (predictor) variables, more comparisons will be possible, and our ability to tease apart—or to better understand—the effects of biology and culture will improve. Systematic comparisons that include biological variables are crucial to this effort. The Melbourne Women's Midlife Health Project, a study that combines traditional surveys with hormonal measures, is an excellent model for researchers in other populations (Dennerstein et al. 1993, 2000).

In addition to thinking about comparable variables, menopause researchers should be aware of advancements in biomedicine's growing ability to predict age at menopause. Women's experience of menopause, along with the ability to plan late childbearing, will change if age at last menstruation can ever be accurately predicted. Moreover, the impermanence of menopause, due to the success of postreproductive pregnancies (using donor eggs) and the possibility of giving birth from cryopreserved ovarian tissue, changes the meaning of the cessation of menstruation. No longer does the cessation of menstruation have to signify the end of fertility.

Comparability

The study of menopause is a multidisciplinary endeavor because there is so much to investigate—the evolution of menopause, age at menopause, variation in symptoms associated with the menopausal transition. One consequence of this multidisciplinarity, however, is a lack of comparability across study samples. Before we can begin to draw firm conclusions about population variation in age at menopause and symptom experience during the menopause transition, we need to improve the comparability of our work. This means comparability of the data collected as well as comparability of the methods used in analysis.

Comparable Variables

We gain different information from cross-species and cross-cultural comparisons of age and symptom experience at menopause than we gain from the best methods applied within one setting. The key to making these comparisons lies in collecting a similar list of variables and carrying out similar analyses. Because of its holism, the biocultural perspective lends itself to collecting a wide range of variables; the focus of other theoretical frameworks restricts the range of variables collected.

For example, if Erin Flanagan and I could have controlled for BMI (kg/m^2) in our study of hot flashes (discussed in Chapter Six) in relation to latitude and temperature, we would have had a much more robust study (Sievert and Flanagan 2005). BMI adds insulation to the body and probably affects the frequency of hot flashes by narrowing the thermoneutral zone. But only a handful of the fifty-six published studies of hot flashes that we used provided an average BMI for the study population. To acquire these data, cultural anthropologists, sociologists, psychologists, epidemiologists, and medical clinicians would need to measure women's height and weight at interview, variables that are quickly and easily collected. The variables carry the same meaning in every cultural context (centimeters and kilograms) and, in the end, the information makes for much stronger comparisons.

This position is not without debate. Melby, Lock, and Kaufert (2005) take the position that "systematization and rigorous analyses are needed, but these will lead us, not to the essence of menopause, but to what is relevant for comparative purposes" (507). These investigators are concerned that standardized questionnaires will impose a universal menopausal framework on women's experiences and, as a consequence, variation will be missed or dismissed. Yet anthropologists should be able to do both—collect comparable data *and* pay attention to the cultural and biological particulars of the population under study.

Simply collecting and publishing the same variables is not meaningful when the characteristics or context of the variables are culture specific. For example, smoking habits, alcohol intake, and educational opportunities differ in culture-specific ways, depending on women's status, roles, and behavioral norms. Therefore, when variables such as these are collected and published, the discussion of context is equally important to help make sense out of contradictory findings.

Comparable Methods

As a reviewer, I often read manuscripts from investigators who submit papers reporting only the mean recalled age at natural menopause. Then, as a researcher, I try to compare that information with published median ages computed by life table analysis. This dilemma could be solved if researchers who publish mean recalled ages at menopause would also publish the median age at natural menopause as computed, relatively simply, by probit analysis. Researchers who have the knowledge base, computer resources, and/or statistical collaboration available to determine age at menopause using life table analysis should also publish probit medians. Then, at the very least, median ages at natural menopause as computed by probit analyses could be compared across all populations.

Researchers across disciplines are often interested in the same phenomenon, but sometimes speak different methodological languages. Particularly in the United States, where researchers are not always mindful that population variation is a global phenomenon, investigators often forget that their work will be used for comparative purposes.

This concern also applies to the problem of where to draw the cutoff between premature ovarian failure and natural menopause. As reviewed in Chapter Four, some populations have a higher proportion of women who experience their last menstrual period prior to age forty. Are all of these women suffering from a pathological state? Probably not. Comparisons of age at menopause across populations need to be clear about where cutoffs have been drawn, and why.

Predicting Age at Menopause

The experience of menopause would change if women knew when in the lifespan it was going to occur. Developing a hormonal test or refining sonographic images to predict age at menopause is an active area of research. As discussed in Chapter One, menopause occurs when a woman's store of ovarian follicles is depleted. As follicle numbers fall, hormone levels change (Rannevik et al. 1995). Elevated levels of FSH early in the menstrual cycle is a commonly used marker of ovarian aging, because elevated FSH levels may indicate a depletion of follicle reserves (Burger et al. 2002; Randolph et al. 2004). This is the basis for the Menocheck test. As discussed in Chapter Two, however, it is difficult for a woman to know whether or not she is nearing her last menstrual period, because hormone levels can vary dramatically every month during perimenopause. Many women have elevated levels of FSH long before they enter perimenopause; therefore FSH levels alone cannot predict a woman's age at menopause.

The rise in FSH levels suggests that FSH is slipping out from under the control of inhibitory hormones, such as inhibin A and inhibin B. As discussed in Chapter Two, inhibin B is produced by developing antral follicles during the reproductive years. Levels rise early in the menstrual cycle, fall before ovulation, and are undetectable in the late menstrual cycle. As women age, inhibin B levels in the early menstrual cycle are diminished; therefore, in addition to levels of FSH, inhibin B can also be used as a marker for the number of follicles in the ovary (Burger et al. 1998; Corson et al. 1999; Danforth et al. 1998; Seifer et al. 1997). But as with FSH, these tests will not tell a woman when her perimenopausal period will end. Antimüllerian hormone, produced in ovarian follicles by granulosa cells, has also been used to assess ovarian reserves, since antimüllerian hormone also declines with increasing female age (De Vet et al. 2002; Van Rooij et al. 2002).

In addition to the measurement of FSH, inhibin B, and antimüllerian hormone, another method being developed to assess ovarian follicular reserves is the measurement of ovarian volume (Flaws et al. 2000; Pavlik et al. 2000). A recent study merged the model of biphasic follicle decline discussed in Chapter One (figure 1.3) with measures of transvaginal sonography. According to Wallace and Kelsey (2004), ovarian volume in women aged twenty-five to fifty-one reflects the number of follicles remaining in the ovary and, by using the model of biphasic follicular decline, age at menopause can be predicted. These investigators assume that follicular decline across the lifespan is biphasic; that variation in age at menopause is due to a difference in follicle number at birth (not rate of atresia); and that menopause occurs at about 50.4 years (on the basis of Treloar 1981). These assumptions are problematic for a number of reasons. First, my colleagues and I have argued that follicular decline is neither biphasic nor more rapid as menopause approaches, but rather occurs at the same rate at the end of the reproductive span (figure 1.4; Leidy et al. 1998). Second, difference in follicle number at birth is one of three parameters determining age at menopause. The other parameters are variation in rates of atresia (demonstrated convincingly in relation to smoking) and variation in the threshold number of oocytes needed to maintain menstrual cyclicity. Third, as Chapter Four illustrated, age at menopause is an aspect of human variation across populations. We are thus still a long way from accurately predicting age at menopause for any individual woman.

Cohort Concerns

As Chapter Three reviewed, a cohort is a group of women born at approximately the same time who share similar health habits, economic stresses, behavioral norms, and diet preferences. The importance of cohort differences was illustrated in relation to hysterectomies (where early cohorts underwent oophorectomies and later cohorts did not). In Chapter Six, the importance of cohort differences was illustrated in relation to ovarian failure due to treatment by chemotherapy and radiation for breast cancers, lymphomas, and other conditions. As cohorts change, questionnaires need to be updated to take into account health habits (for example, marijuana use) or chemical/radiation exposures not common in earlier cohorts. It isn't that women in earlier cohorts didn't use marijuana, but marijuana use was less prevalent. Similarly, it isn't that women in earlier cohorts didn't experience premenopausal breast cancer or lymphoma, but women are now more likely to survive and to be experiencing the effects of chemotherapy, which include an earlier age at menopause and elevated symptom frequency.

The Impermanence of Menopause

Two areas of clinical research are contributing to the reversal of menopause. The first is the potential for continued ovarian function through auto-ovarian grafts. The second is postmenopausal assisted pregnancy using donor eggs.

Fertility is a major concern for women who have survived cancer during childhood or during the early reproductive years (Blumenfeld 2002; Revel and Laufer 2002). Researchers have been working to preserve fertility and ovarian function during chemotherapy (Blumenfeld 2002) or to restore fertility to women after the damage has been done. One goal has been to remove, preserve, and reimplant a woman's own ovarian tissue.

Attempts at ovarian tissue cryopreservation and transplantation date back to the 1950s. Initial studies were disappointing because glycerol, the only available cryoprotectant, was ineffective for cryopreservation of human oocytes and ovarian tissue (reviewed in Oktay 2001). With the advent of more effective cryoprotectants, animal studies were repeated and successful deliveries were reported in a number of species (Candy et al. 2000; Gosden et al. 1994; Sztein et al. 1998). In humans, resumption of ovarian endocrine function was demonstrated (Oktay and Karlikaya 2000; Radford et al. 2001), and an embryo following subcutaneous transplantation of cryopreserved ovarian tissue was reported (Oktay and Sonmezer 2004).

Donnez et al. (2004) reported a live birth after the transplantation of cryopreserved ovarian tissue. In this case, five biopsy samples were taken from the ovary of a twenty-five-year-old woman with Hodgkin's lymphoma. The ovarian tissue was frozen. Following chemotherapy, the woman experienced ovarian failure as assessed by elevated levels of FSH and LH and low levels of estrogen. To reimplant the ovarian tissue, years later, a peritoneal window was created very close to the ovaries and, seven days later, thawed ovarian tissue was pushed into the peritoneal space. Follicular development and menstrual cyclicity returned. Conception took place spontaneously following ovulation, nine months after the reimplantation. The pregnancy resulted in the live birth of a healthy girl.

Cornell University's Weill Medical College in New York stores frozen ovarian tissue from about sixty women, and several other fertility clinics offer similar services for fees of $6,000 or more. "If the ovarian-tissue technique is perfected, it could find other uses, doctors predict. For instance, some women may seek to freeze parts of their ovaries while they are young in order to extend the age at which they can reproduce" (Regalado 2004:B3).

In a second area of research, biomedical researchers have been working to extend the length of the reproductive period by assisting peri- or postmenopausal women carry pregnancies to term (Antinori et al. 1993; Sauer, Paulson, and Lobo 1992). From a lifespan perspective, older women accumulate difficulties that may preclude late childbearing. These difficulties include endometriosis, tubal obstruction subsequent to pelvic inflammatory disease, the production of sperm antibodies, and the side effects of contraceptives. In addition, premature ovarian failure (POF) or natural menopause brings about an end to childbearing. All of these problems can now be addressed, to varying extents, through infertility treatment (Benshushan and Schenker 1993; Bustillo et al. 1984).

While in vitro fertilization (IVF) success rates are very low for women older than forty using their own eggs (Chetkowski et al. 1991; Meldrum 1993; Sauer, Paulson, and Lobo 1992), oocyte donation has become a successful "treatment" for menopause in women older than fifty (Antinori et al. 1993; Sauer et al. 1993) or even sixty years of age (Antinori et al. 1995; Kolata 1997; Paulson et al. 1997). For example, in one study sample, women seeking egg donation ranged from fifty to fifty-nine years of age (mean 52.2 years). Their husbands ranged from twenty-seven to seventy years of age (mean 47.8 years). Of fourteen couples assisted, eight women had never had a child (Sauer et al. 1993).

Ethical concerns specific to postmenopausal pregnancy revolve around the health of the woman and the future of the children. With age, there is an increased risk of obstetric complication such as pregnancy-induced hypertension, gestational diabetes, and placenta previa; maternal mortality; an increased rate of chromosomal abnormalities in the oocytes; and an increased risk of fetal deaths (Berkowitz et al. 1990; Breart 1997; Buehler et al. 1986; Cnattingius et al. 1992; Fretts et al. 1995; Friede et al. 1988; Kirz et al. 1985; Lansac 1995; Maroulis 1991; Meldrum 1993; Naeye 1983; Richardson and Nelson 1990; Schmidt-Sarosi 1998; Stein 1985). In seventeen viable pregnancies detailed by Sauer et al. (1995), nine were multiple gestations (six twins, one triplet, and two quadruplets selectively terminated to twins), and complications were described in eight patients (including gestational hypertension, gestational diabetes, and preeclampsia). Regarding the health of the children, worries include whether or not aging mothers can cope with the physical demands of childrearing (Belkin 1997), but this ignores the fact that children have often been raised by grandparents (remember the grandmother hypothesis for the evolution of menopause). Others worry that older mothers will leave orphans (Benshushan and Schenker 1993). In response, it is pointed out that the expected lifespan has never been longer (Mori 1994) and "there was no talk of orphans when only men could conceive into their seventies or older" (Edwards 1993:1543).

In Conclusion

The wide range in age at menopause within any one population is not easy to explain. To some extent, age at menopause is related to genetic inheritance (Snieder, MacGregor, and Spector 1998). However, menopause occurs after fifty years of living, or after the effects of gestation, infancy, childhood, adolescence, and reproduction have taken their toll on the ovarian follicles. Because human females store their eggs in their ovaries for all of that time, the eggs are affected by biobehavioral factors such as smoking habits (Mattison et al. 1989)—perhaps of their mothers as well as of their own. A lifespan approach allows the researcher to investigate variation in age at menopause across, as well as within, populations.

One general observation can be made about age at menopause: variables associated with age at menopause demonstrate similar within-population relationships across cultures. For example, smoking is associated with an earlier age at menopause in the United States (Brambilla and McKinlay 1989), Mexico (Sievert and Hautaniemi 2003), Finland (Luoto, Kaprio, and Uutela 1994), Italy (Parazzini, Negri, and La Vecchia 1992), and Australia (Do et al. 1998). This association suggests that the effect of smoking on age at menopause is primarily biological; that is, smoking affects the ovaries directly or indirectly and shortens the reproductive span.

Variables associated with within-population variation in age at menopause, however, do not necessarily explain across-population variation in age at menopause. For example, if smoking is associated with an earlier age at menopause, one might think that populations with high rates of female smoking would have the earliest ages at menopause, but this is not the case. In fact, the opposite is often true. Part of the explanation is that smoking is not just a "biological" variable. In the United States, smoking is more common among women of lower socioeconomic status. In Mexico, smoking is more common among women of higher socioeconomic status. Differential access to health care, diet, and other basics may also affect variation in age at menopause. Whenever we try to understand the relationship between even the most seemingly straightforward variables and age at menopause, it is important to step back and ask about correlated variables in the culture of which the study participants are part.

If determining reasons for variation in age at menopause is difficult, Chapters Five and Six demonstrated that understanding variation in symptom frequencies is even more so. This difficulty stems in part, from the many interacting variables that need to be pulled apart. In addition, variables associated with symptom experience at menopause do not necessarily demonstrate similar within-population relationships across cultures.

The study of menopause has never been more interesting. Researchers argue passionately in defense of the grandmother hypothesis to explain the evolution of menopause. With more comparable data, we should be able to draw cross-population conclusions about variation in age at menopause. As it is, we know more than ever before about the heritability of menopause and the effect of health habits on ovarian stores. The cause of hot flashes is understood better than ever before (that is, in terms of the narrowing of the thermoneutral zone), but why one woman suffers while another woman can wear turtleneck sweaters remains a mystery.

In addition to the biological advances that have taken place in recent years (such as the discovery of inhibin A and inhibin B, the use of antimüllerian hormone as a marker of ovarian reserve, the better understanding of the role of neurotransmitters at the level of the hypothalamus), a better appreciation of the role of attitudes and social stress has also developed. At the same time, in the cultural arena of biomedicine, the often unquestioned dominance of hormone therapy as a treatment for all menopausal women has come to an end. Medical doctors are struggling to know what to prescribe. To make things more complicated, medical advances have resulted in postmenopausal pregnancies and a birth following the cryopreservation of ovarian tissue.

Menopause is a species-level trait. It demonstrates impressive population-level variation that, ultimately, affects individual lives. It is the anecdotal evidence that reminds me that all of this excitement—evolutionary argument, statistical analysis, and biomedical advance—is more than an academic exercise. As part of a pilot project in Hilo, Hawaii, in the summer of 2005, we recruited a soft-spoken, premenopausal nurse to wear our ambulatory hot flash monitor. She returned the monitor and said simply that she thought she had one hot flash, so she pressed the marker buttons. We thanked her and went back to the university to download the data, then returned the next day with the output and a box of chocolate. The monitor had measured the conductance of electricity from one electrode to another across her upper chest. The data output showed a straight line for a couple of hours, and then a dramatic increase in the conductance of electricity (due to sweating) that corresponded with the timing of her hot flash. She studied the graphed results, and said simply, "So it's not in my head!"

No, it's not in our heads. In this text I have not minimized the discomforts associated with menopause, and I have emphasized that hormonal changes can only explain part of the story. Perhaps, if I had not worked for so long in Mexico, I would try to spin hot flashes into positive "power surges," as some observers do. However, I have met some terrifically unhappy women who cannot sleep through the night because they have to open windows, close windows, turn on fans, turn off fans, and change sheets to cope with their sweating. They have, consequently or coincidentally, stopped sleeping with their husbands. Sometimes it is an angry husband who wants to speak to me, when I want to interview his wife. I have met men who tell me they want to kill their wives, as if that's an understandable reaction on their part.

A biocultural perspective, coupled with a lifespan approach, provides a way to understand which aspects of age at menopause and symptom experience are genetic, which fall under hormonal control, and which are open to environmental influence. A better understanding of the menopause transition within and across populations can only improve the circumstances of women's health, in the broadest of all possible senses.

NOTES

CHAPTER ONE   INTRODUCTION

1. As Mary Pavelka explained to me, identifying female macaques who have actually stopped reproducing and are truly in a postreproductive stage of life is difficult. Often researchers treat the time lag between the birth of the last infant and the mother's death as a postreproductive period, but it is not necessarily so: the mother may have simply died during a regular interval between infants, and would have been able to have more had she lived. To avoid this problem, Pavelka and Fedigan only considered females to be postreproductive if they lived for a "long time" without having an infant before they died. By a long time, they mean that the females' time without having a baby was significantly longer than any previous gap between births. For each female, Pavelka and Fedigan looked at all of the intervals between infants and took the average, and then to this value added two standard deviations. Thus they classified a female as postreproductive only if she lived significantly longer than her own mean lifetime interbirth interval, without having a baby, before she died. This method reduces the likelihood of categorizing females as reproductively terminated simply because they died before having another baby (personal communication).

2. The perineum is the area between the genitalia and the anus that swells when the female chimpanzee is fertile.

3. "Natural menopause" excludes menopause due to hysterectomy (which also results in a permanent cessation of menstruation) or chemotherapy (which can result in the loss of ovarian follicular activity).

4. The researchers note that blood samples for hormone levels were taken from premenopausal women at different phases of the menstrual cycle as it was not possible to synchronize the sampling of many women to a particular day of the cycle. This was particularly true as the frequency of irregular bleeding intervals increased. The authors go on to say, however, that "the large number of samples in the premenopausal period from most of the women permitted, when appropriate, analysis of data according to the various phases of the menstrual cycle" (Rannevik et al. 1995:105).

5. Because the standard deviation includes most but not all of the variation measured, a few women will actually have FSH levels lower than $1 \mu g/l$ and some will have levels higher than $4 \mu g/l$.

6. Although the word "symptom" is indicative of biomedicine's tendency to pathologize menopause, alternative words such as "complaints," "discomforts," or "indications" can minimize the severity of some women's experiences. In this book I use the word "symptom" to avoid minimizing what, for some women, is a very difficult experience.

At the same time, I recognize that many women have no "symptoms" at all, or very mild discomforts.

7. Change in the regularity of menstruation (having periods closer or farther apart) is used to classify women as perimenopausal, whereas volume of blood flow (heavy or light) is not. However, many women may have either lighter or heavier periods as they approach menopause.

8. This conventional wisdom was called into question by Baker (1986) in a discussion of prosimians (small-bodied primates). Some prosimians apparently have "nests" of developing eggs in their ovaries after birth. More recently, Johnson et al. (2004) demonstrated that mice are capable of producing eggs after birth. The implications of these discoveries for humans are not yet known.

9. Although physicians were mistaken on this point, there are plenty of other reasons to encourage women to avoid having children at older maternal ages, such as an increase in risk of miscarriage and an increase in the risk of bearing a child with chromosomal abnormalities (Roberts and O'Neill 1995; Wood 1994).

10. I am grateful to my colleague Laurie Godfrey for pointing this out.

11. The political-economic perspective has a long, rich history in the biological anthropology of Mexico.

12. This is an "etic" approach in the sense that standardized assessments are used to collect factors such as symptoms or attitudes. These assessments are replicable. Emic data, on the other hand, include understanding the intentions and meanings associated with particular behavior patterns within a local context. A meaning-centered approach is culture-specific and far less comparable across populations.

13. I would argue that the highest frequency of hot flashes among married women without children reflects a sadness related to not fulfilling cultural expectations. When women were asked to describe a woman of menopausal age as a "success" or a "failure," women in Puebla who had not had children would often choose the word failure and sometimes cry at that point while explaining that they had been unable to become pregnant. From a biocultural perspective, this is similar to what Dressler (1996) measures—the discrepancy between cultural expectation and behavior (here, the behavior of giving birth). However, while giving birth is a biological event, it can also be considered an artifact of culture, since access to medical services, for example, influences the biological outcome.

14. Reproductive span was computed as age at menopause minus age at menarche.

15. This figure is similar to the frequency of tubal ligation (44 percent) for all of Mexico (CONAPO 2004).

CHAPTER TWO   THE BIOLOGICAL BASIS OF MENOPAUSE

1. It was discovered in the mid-1990s that there are actually two types of estrogen receptors, ER-α and ER-β. Although they both respond to the same hormones, they are differentially distributed in the body. For example, ER-β receptors are more prevalent in certain areas of the brain and cardiovascular system (Enmark et al. 1997). This pattern of distribution has been important for targeting the treatment of osteoporosis without affecting other tissues like the endometrium (Fuleihan 1997).

2. Pulse frequency is the number of pulses that occur within a given period of time. Pulse amplitude is the maximum value of a pulse. Think of frequencies as going across time and think of amplitudes as going up and down (that is, as periodic variations in hormonal secretion).

3. In contrast, in old female rodents the hypothalamus is the source of reproductive function and decline. Unlike humans, the pituitary and ovaries remain functional in old female rats as demonstrated by the transplantation of these organs from old rats into young rats. The decline in dopamine and norepinephrine appears to be mainly responsible for the loss of estrous cycles in aging female rats (Meites and Lu 1994).

4. To compute your own BMI, multiply your weight in pounds by 704.5 and divide by your height squared (height in inches × height in inches). If you weigh 145 pounds and are 5′7″ tall, your BMI is 145 × 704.5 = 102152.5, divided by 67 × 67 or 22.8.

5. However, they also demonstrate a very low probability that a woman will die within the first five years after a birth until she is very old.

6. This argument assumes a maximum lifespan potential of fifty (similar to current chimpanzees) prior to the selection for a longer postreproductive life. Thus, the argument goes, in our species the body lived on, but the ovaries ceased functioning at fifty.

CHAPTER THREE   METHODS OF STUDY

1. The Human Relations Area Files were established in 1937 by the Institute of Human Relations at Yale University under the direction of George P. Murdock and, after 1945, Clellan S. Ford. The goal was "to organize in readily accessible form the available data on a statistically representative sample of all known cultures—primitive, historical, and contemporary—for the purpose of testing cross-cultural generalizations, revealing deficiencies in the descriptive literature, and directing corrective field work" (Murdock et al. 1982:xxi).

2. In Berglund's analysis menopause was understood in symbolic terms in association with the cult of the ancestors. Among the Zulu, the departed ancestors, or "shades," were thought to exist in dreams and cause physical manifestations such as menstrual blood. A woman had her father's shades in her womb, causing the blood to come regularly each month. Old women who could no longer bear children were thought to have been abandoned by their lineage shades. "They [the shades] see that she is drying. So they leave her. The blood becomes less and less. . . . That is when they commence becoming like men" (Berglund 1976:121).

3. Later researchers used different (life table) statistical techniques and limited the same sample to women who experienced menopause between the ages of 44 and 56 years to achieve an estimated mean age at natural menopause of 50.5 years (Whelan et al. 1990).

4. As will be discussed further in Chapter Six, lack of interest in menopause did not extend to the medical profession; physicians had been writing articles and books about menopause since the mid-1800s (Lock and Kaufert 2001). By the 1940s, menopause was beginning to be medically managed with estrogen (Lock 1993). By the 1960s, when the first large-scale studies of age at menopause were being conducted in the Netherlands and the United States, menopause was being widely treated with what was then called estrogen replacement therapy (ERT) as a way to keep women young (Wilson 1966).

5. Despite Whitehead's (1994) claim, Jaszmann was hardly the first to suggest a connection between psychological symptoms and ovarian status. "Involutional melancholia" was a depressive disorder attributed to the menopause transition by Kraeplin in 1896, and maintained as a diagnostic category in the Diagnostic and Statistical Manual of the American Psychiatric Association until 1979 (H. Ford 1975). Involutional melancholia is discussed further in Chapter Five.

6. In a snowball approach participants are selected through networks of friends, relatives, and acquaintances. A participant is asked to name other people who might be interested in participating in the study. Then those people are asked for names, and the list snowballs from there. The limitation of this method is that it produces a bias toward people who share similar characteristics, such as place of residence or socioeconomic status. This may not be a problem if the study focuses on ethnic differences in symptom experience, as in the SWAN study. However, it must be kept in mind that the snowball technique cannot produce a random sample within a particular ethnic group.

7. Perhaps a small point, but it may be helpful to note that the British prefer to refer to hot "flushes" while Americans prefer to experience hot "flashes."

8. Beginning in 1994, I have lived in Puebla for periods ranging from one to eight weeks each summer and, when possible, for one to three weeks in January as well.

9. According to the packaging, Mensifem is a nonhormonal treatment that contributes to emotional balance and relieves the symptoms of menopause such as hot flashes and sweating.

10. The Kupperman/Blatt Menopausal Index was developed to facilitate, for example, a comparison of the efficacy of vitamin E (50–100 mg daily), ethinyl estradiol (0.05 mg daily), conjugated equine estrogens (1.25 mg daily), phenobarbital (15 mg three times a day), and placebo (1 tablet daily) in treating menopausal symptoms. Note that the dose of conjugated equine estrogens (Premarin) was double that prescribed today. The index showed that the two estrogen preparations were equally effective, associated with an excellent response in 66.5 percent of the patients treated, compared with 24 percent of patients taking phenobarbital, 13 percent of patients taking vitamin E, and 16 percent of patients taking placebo (Blatt, Wiesbader, and Kupperman 1953).

11. I am always surprised by the number of women who undergo a hysterectomy and do not know if they still have their ovaries or not. For example, in a clinical study of hot flashes carried out Puebla, Mexico, seven women thought that their ovaries had been removed during a hysterectomy. To the contrary, blood tests showed that they were still producing premenopausal levels of estrogen (Sievert et al. 2002), which indicated that their ovaries were still there.

12. In Mexico, one traditional way believed to avoid hysterectomies following the diagnosis of a fibroid tumor is to buy a special clay and place a tortilla-shaped patty on the lower abdomen every night. It is thought that the clay draws out the toxins and shrinks the tumor.

13. Uterine artery embolization involves placing a small incision in the inner thigh to thread a small catheter from the groin to the tiny blood vessels that nourish the fibroid tumor. Microparticles are injected into the blood vessels to act like little plugs. The idea is to shrink the fibroid without damaging the uterus.

CHAPTER FOUR   AGE AT MENOPAUSE

1. Alternatively, it may be more correct to say that an underlying mechanism associated with both the trait of interest (say, number of births) and age at menopause exerts its effect on age at menopause some time prior to the cessation of menstruation. Some traits (such as pregnancy) probably do not have a direct effect on age at menopause.

2. Although it is a fun hypothesis, I have never collected adequate sample sizes to test the effects of playing with X-ray machines in shoe stores on age at menopause.

3. In humans, genes are arranged along 46 chromosomes—44 are autosomes and 2 are sex chromosomes. Women are 46,XX. Men are 46,XY. Women with Turner's syndrome have only 45 chromosomes (45,X).

4. Even so, distributions in age at menopause and in ages of menstruating women are rarely published. See Stanford et al. (1987) for an exception.

5. Some people use the term "secular" to describe unidirectional changes that are visible across one generation, or even ten years, but Barry Bogin suggests using the term "time trends" to describe change across shorter spans of time (personal communication).

6. The Cox model gives the likelihood that women in a particular exposure category (such as women who smoke) will be menopausal relative to women in another category (such as women who do not smoke) adjusted for other exposure variables (such as history of pregnancy) (Cramer and Xu 1996). According to Susan Hautaniemi Leonard, in Cox proportional hazards regression the dependent variable is the probability that an event will occur to an individual at a given time. For more details, see Sievert and Hautaniemi (2003).

7. Some women elaborated on their responses to the structured food list to explain that even though they came from a "humble" background, they had access to good food because, for example, their family had a cow or their grandfather was a butcher. Childhood food intake was thus dissociated from social class for many women.

8. Interestingly, these measures of mental ability were not highly correlated with educational attainment.

CHAPTER FIVE   THE DISCOMFORTS OF MENOPAUSE

1. In Hong Kong perimenopausal women reported a higher frequency of depression (29 percent) compared with premenopausal (17 percent) or postmenopausal women (11 percent), $p < .01$. In Malaysia, postmenopausal women reported the highest frequency of depression (35 percent) compared with premenopausal (21 percent) and perimenopausal (11 percent) women, $p < .01$ (Boulet et al. 1994).

2. More specifically, it is the distal vagina, close to the opening, that is rich in estrogen receptors. The same is not true of the inner vagina, because the cells of the inner vagina have a different embryological origin. Vaginal dryness, then, most severely affects the tissue at the vaginal entrance.

CHAPTER SIX   HOT FLASHES

1. Physiological studies show no change in blood pressure during a hot flash. Heart rate does increase, but blood pressure stays the same.

2. My thanks to Elena Brown for this diagram.

3. HT does reduce bone loss, but is no longer recommended as a preventative for coronary heart disease in women of any age or for the primary prevention of dementia in women older than sixty-five (Manson et al. 2003; Shumaker et al. 2003; Writing Group 2002; and the October 2004 Position Statement of the North American Menopause Society).

4. Tamoxifen can function as an estrogen agonist in other parts of the body, increasing estrogen in, for example, the vagina and endometrium.

REFERENCES

Abdalla, H. I., Baber, R., Kirkland, A., Leonard, T., Power, M., and Studd, J.W.W. 1990. A report on 100 cycles of oocyte donation: factors affecting the outcome. *Human Reproduction* 5:1018–1022.

Abe, T., Suzuki, M., Wada, Y., Yamaya, Y., and Moritsuka, T. 1985. Clinical and endocrinological features of statistical clusters of women with climacteric symptoms. *Tohoku Journal of Experimental Medicine* 146:59–68.

Adlercreutz, H., Hamalainen, E., Gorbach, G., and Goldin, B. 1992. Dietary phytoestrogens and the menopause in Japan. *Lancet* 339:1233.

Agoestina, T., and van Keep, P. A. 1984. The climacteric in Bandung, West Java province, Indonesia. *Maturitas* 6:327–333.

Alcorn, G. T., and Robinson, E. S. 1983. Germ-cell development in female pouch young of the tammar wallaby *(Macropus eugenii). Journal of Reproduction and Fertility* 67(2):319–325.

Aldous, M. B., and Edmonson, M. B. 1993. Maternal age at first childbirth and risk of low birth weight and preterm delivery in Washington State. *Journal of the American Medical Association* 270:2574–2577.

Alexander, R. D. 1974. The evolution of social behavior. *Annual Review of Ecology and Systematics* 5:325–383.

Alper, M. M., and Garner, P. R. 1985. Premature ovarian failure and its relationship to autoimmune disease. *Obstetrics and Gynecology* 66:27–30.

Althaus, F. 1994. Both biological and motivational factors may play a role in higher hysterectomy risk after sterilization. *Family Planning Perspectives* 26(1):44–45.

Altorki, S. 1986. *Women in Saudi Arabia: Ideology and Behavior among the Elite.* New York: Columbia University Press.

American College of Physicians. 1992. Guidelines for counseling postmenopausal women about preventive hormone therapy. *Annals of Internal Medicine* 117:1048–1051.

Amundsen, D. W., and Diers, C. J. 1973. The age of menopause in Medieval Europe. *Human Biology* 45(4):605–612.

Anderson, D. J. 2000. Immunologic aspects of menopause. In R. A. Lobo, J. Kelsey, and R. Marcus, eds., *Menopause: Biology and Pathology,* 353–357. New York: Academic Press.

Anderson, D., Yoshizawa, T., Atogami, F., Hiraishi, M., and Gollschewski, S. 2002. The relationship between menopausal symptoms and menopausal status in Australian and Japanese women. Poster presentation, thirteenth annual meeting of the North American Menopause Society, Chicago, October 3–5.

Anderson, D., Yoshizawa, T., Gollschewski, S., Atogami, F., and Courtney, M. 2004. Menopause in Australia and Japan: the effects of country of residence on menopausal status and menopausal symptoms. *Climacteric* 7(2):165–174.

Antinori, S., Versaci, C., Hossein Gholami, G., Panci, C., and Caffa, B. 1993. Oocyte donation in menopausal women. *Human Reproduction* 8:1487–1490.

Antinori, S., Versaci, C., Panci, C., Caffa, B., and Hossein Gholami, G. 1995. Fetal and maternal morbidity and mortality in menopausal women aged 45–63 years. *Human Reproduction* 10(2):464–469.

Aréchiga, J., Monsalve, T., Prado, C., Cantó, M., Carmenate, M., and Martínez, A. 2000. Doing what comes naturally: women in transition, menopause, and body composition in different populations. Poster presentation, eleventh annual meeting of the North American Menopause Society, Orlando, FL., Sept. 7–9.

Asch, R. H., Smith, C. G., Siler-Khodr, T. M., and Pauerstein, C. J. 1981. Effects of Δ^9-tetrahydrocannabinol during the follicular phase of the rhesus monkey *(Macaca mulatta)*. *Journal of Clinical Endocrinology and Metabolism* 52:50–55.

Austad, S. N. 1997. Postreproductive survival. In K. W. Wachter, and C. E. Finch, eds., *Between Zeus and the Salmon: the Biodemography of Longevity,* 161–174. Washington, DC: National Academy Press.

Avis, N. E., Brambilla, D., McKinlay, S. M., and Vass, K. 1994. A longitudinal analysis of the association between menopause and depression. *Annals of Epidemiology* 4:214–220.

Avis, N. E., Crawford, S. L., and McKinlay, S. M. 1997. Psychosocial, behavioral, and health factors related to menopause symptomatology. *Women's Health* 3:103–120.

Avis, N. E., Kaufert, P. A., Lock, M., McKinlay, S. M., and Vass, K. 1993. The evolution of menopausal symptoms. *Baillière's Clinical Endocrinology and Metabolism* 7:17–32.

Avis, N. E., and McKinlay, S. M. 1991. A longitudinal analysis of women's attitudes towards the menopause: results from the Massachusetts Women's Health Study. *Maturitas* 13:65–79.

Avis, N. E., Ory, M., Matthews, K. A., Schocken, M., Bromberger, J., and Colvin, A. 2003. Health-related quality of life in a multiethnic sample of middle-aged women: Study of Women's Health Across the Nation (SWAN). *Medical Care* 41(11):1262–1276.

Avis, N. E., Stellato, R., Crawford, S., Bromberger, J., Ganz, P., Cain, V., and Kagawa-Singer, M. 2001. Is there a menopausal syndrome? Menopausal status and symptoms across racial/ethnic groups. *Social Science and Medicine* 52(3):345–356.

Bachmann, G. A., and Nevadunsky, N. S. 2000. Diagnosis and treatment of atrophic vaginitis. *American Family Physician* 61:3090–3096.

Backett-Milburn, K., Parry, O., and Mauthner, N. 2000. "I'll worry about that when it comes along": osteoporosis, a meaningful issue for women at mid-life? *Health Education Research* (15):153–162.

Backstrom, C. T., McNeilly, A., Leask, R. M., and Bird, D. T. 1982. Pulsatile secretion of LH, FSH, prolactin, estradiol, and progesterone during the human menstrual cycle. *Clinical Endocrinology* 17:29–42.

Baker, P. T. 1984. The adaptive limits of human populations. *Man* 19:1–14.

Baker, T. G. 1986. Gametogenesis. In W. R. Dukelow, and J. Erwin, eds., *Comparative Primate Biology,* vol. 3: *Reproduction and Development,* 195–213. New York: Alan R. Liss.

Ballinger, C. B. 1990. Psychiatric aspects of the menopause. *British Journal of Psychiatry* 156:773–787.

Ballinger, C. B., Browning, M.C.K., and Smith, A.H.W. 1987. Hormone profiles and psychological symptoms in peri-menopausal women. *Maturitas* 9:235–251.

Ballinger, S. E. 1985. Psychosocial stress and symptoms of menopause: a comparative study of menopause clinic patients and non-patients. *Maturitas* 7:315–327.

Baltes, P. B., and Schaie, K. W. 1973. On life-span developmental research paradigms: retrospects and prospects. In P. B. Baltes, and K. W. Schaie, eds., *Life-Span Developmental Psychology*, 365–431. New York: Academic Press.

Barker, K.J.P. 1998. *Mothers, Babies, and Disease in Later Life*. 2nd ed. New York: Churchill Livingstone.

Barnett, E. A. 1988. La edad critica: The positive experience of menopause in a small Peruvian town. In P. Whelehan, ed., *Women and Health: Cross-Cultural Perspectives*, 40–54. Granby, MA: Bergin and Garvey.

Baron, J. A., and Greenberg, E. R. 1987. Cigarette smoking and estrogen-related disease in women. In M. J. Rosenberg, ed., *Smoking and Reproductive Health*, 149–160. Littleton, MA: PSG Publishing.

Baron, J. A., La Vecchia, C., and Levi, F. 1990. The anti-estrogenic effect of cigarette smoking in women. *American Journal of Obstetrics and Gynecology* 162:502–514.

Barroso Benítez, A. 2003. Envejecimiento reproductor en mujeres españolas desde una perspectiva ecológica y de ciclo vital. Ph.D. diss., Department of Biology, Anthropology Unit, Universidad Autonoma de Madrid.

Bart, P. B. 1969. Why women's status changes in middle age: the turns of the social ferris wheel. *Sociological Symposium* 3:1–18.

———. 1971. Depression in middle-aged women. In V. Fornick, and B. Moran, eds., *Woman in Sexist Society*, 99–117. New York: Basic Books.

Basson, R. 2000. The female sexual response: a different model. *Journal of Sex and Marital Therapy* 26:51–65.

Bean, J. A., Leeper, J. D., Wallace, R. B., Sherman, B. M., and Jagger, H. 1979. Variations in the reporting of menstrual histories. *American Journal of Epidemiology* 109(2):181–185.

Belkin, L. 1997. Pregnant with complications. *New York Times Magazine*, Oct. 26:34–39, 48–49.

Bell, M. L. 1995. Attitudes toward menopause among Mexican-American women. *Health Care for Women International* 16:425–435.

Bell, S. E. 1987. Changing ideas: the medicalization of menopause. *Social Science and Medicine* 24(6):535–542.

Benjamin, C. 1966. Ideas of time in the history of philosophy. In J. T. Fraser, ed., *The Voices of Time: A Cooperative Survey of Man's Views of Time as Expressed by the Sciences and by the Humanities*, 3–30. New York: Braziller.

Bennett, G. W., and Whitehead, S. A. 1983. *Mammalian Neuroendocrinology*. New York: Oxford University Press.

Benshushan, A., and Schenker, J. G. 1993. Ovum donation—an overview. *Journal of Assisted Reproduction and Genetics* 10(2):105–111.

Bentley, G. R., Paine, R. R., and Boldsen, J. L. 2001. Fertility changes with the prehistoric transition to agriculture: perspectives from reproductive ecology and paleodemography. In P. T. Ellison, ed., *Reproductive Ecology and Human Evolution*, 203–231. New York: Aldine de Gruyter.

Berg, G., Gottqall, T., Hammer, M., and Lindgren, R. 1988. Climacteric symptoms among women aged 60–62 in Linksping, Sweden, in 1986. *Maturitas* 10:193–199.

Berglund, A.-I. 1976. *Zulu Thought-Patterns and Symbolism*. Uppsala: Swedish Institute of Missionary Research.

Berkowitz, G. S., Skovron, M. L., Lapinski, R. H., and Berkowitz, R. L. 1990. Delayed childbearing and the outcome of pregnancy. *New England Journal of Medicine* 322(10):659–664.

Bernis, C. 2001. Ecología del envejecimiento reproductor. In C. Bernis Carro, R. López Giménez, C. Prado Martínez, and J. Sebastián Herranz, eds., *Salud y género: la salud de la mujer en el umbral del siglo XXI,* 129–143. Instituto Universitario de Estudios de la Mujer, XIII Jornadas de Investigación Interdisciplinarias.

Bernstein, S. J., Fiske, M. E., McGlynn, E. A., and Gifford, D. S. 1997. *Hysterectomy: A Review of the Literature on Indications, Effectiveness, and Risks.* Santa Monica, CA: RAND.

Bernstein, S. J., McGlynn, E. A., Kamberg, C. J., Chassin, M. R., Goldberg, G. A., Siu, A. L., and Brook, R. H. 1992. *Hysterectomy: A Literature Review and Ratings of Appropriateness.* Santa Monica, CA: RAND.

Beyene, Y. 1986. Cultural significance and physiological manifestations of menopause: a biocultural analysis. *Culture, Medicine and Psychiatry* 10:47–71.

———. 1989. *From Menarche to Menopause: Reproductive Histories of Peasant Women in Two Cultures.* Albany: State University of New York Press.

Beyene, Y., and Martin, M. C. 2001. Menopausal experiences and bone density of Mayan women in Yucatan, Mexico. *American Journal of Human Biology* 13:505–511.

Bharadwaj, J. A., Kendurkar, S. M., and Vaidya, P. R. 1983. Age and symptomatology of menopause in Indian women. *Journal of Postgraduate Medicine* 29(4):218–222.

Bickell, N. A., Earp, J. A., Garrett, J. M., and Evans, A. T. 1994. Gynecologists' sex, clinical beliefs, and hysterectomy rates. *American Journal of Public Health* 84:1649–1652.

Birchfield, P. C. 2001. Osteoarthritis overview. *Geriatric Nursing* 22(3):124–131.

Blatt, M. H., Wiesbader, H., and Kupperman, H. 1953. Vitamin E and climacteric syndrome: failure of effective control as measured by menopausal index. *AMA Archives of Internal Medicine* 91:792–799.

Block, E. 1952. Quantitative morphological investigations of the follicular system in women. II. Variations at different ages. *Acta Anatomica* 14:108–123.

———. 1953. A quantitative morphological investigation of the follicular system in newborn female infants. *Acta Anatomica* 17:201–206.

Blumenfeld, Z. 2002. Preservation of fertility and ovarian function and minimalization of chemotherapy associated gonadotoxicity and premature ovarian failure: the role of inhibin-A and -B as markers. *Molecular and Cellular Endocrinology* 187(1–2):93–105.

Bogin, B. 1998. Milk and human development: an essay on the "milk hypothesis." *Antropologia Portuguesa* 15:23–36.

———. 1999. *Patterns of Human Growth.* 2nd ed. New York: Cambridge University Press.

Bogin, B., and Loucky, J., 1997. Political economy and physical growth of Guatemala Maya children living in the United States. *American Journal of Physical Anthropology* 102:17–32.

Bogin, B., and Smith, B. H. 1996. Evolution of the human life cycle. *American Journal of Human Biology* 8:703–716.

Boulet, M. J., Oddens, B. J., Lehert, P., Vemer, H. M., and Visser, A. 1994. Climacteric and menopause in seven south-east Asian countries. *Maturitas* 19(3):157–176.

Bowles, C. 1986. Measure of attitude toward menopause using the semantic differential model. *Nursing Research* 35(2):81–85.

Bradsher, J. E., and McKinlay, S. M. 2000. Distinguishing the effects of age from those of menopause. In R. A. Lobo, J. Kelsey, and R. Marcus, eds., *Menopause: Biology and Pathobiology,* 203–211. New York: Academic Press.

Brambilla, D., and McKinlay, S. M. 1989. A prospective study of factors affecting age at menopause. *Journal of Clinical Epidemiology* 42:1031–1039.

Brand, P. C., and Lehert, P. H. 1978. A new way of looking at environmental variables that may affect the age at menopause. *Maturitas* 1:121–132.

Breart, G. 1997. Delayed childbearing. *European Journal of Obstetrics, Gynecology, and Reproductive Biology* 75(1):71–73.

Brett, K. M., Marsh, J. V., and Madans, J. H. 1997. Epidemiology of hysterectomy in the United States: demographic and reproductive factors in a nationally representative sample. *Journal of Women's Health* 6(3):309–316.

Brettell, C. B. 2002. Gendered lives: transitions and turning points in personal, family, and historical time. *Current Anthropology* 43(supp.):S45–S61.

Brim, O. G., and Kagan, J. 1980. Constancy and change: a view of the issues. In O. G. Brim, and J. Kagan, eds., *Constancy and Change in Human Development*, 1–25. Cambridge, MA: Harvard University Press.

Bromberger, J. T., Harlow, S., Avis, N., Kravitz, H. M., and Cordal, A. 2004. Racial/ethnic differences in the prevalence of depressive symptoms among middle-aged women: The Study of Women's Health Across the Nation (SWAN). *American Journal of Public Health* 94(8):1378–1385.

Brooks, J. D., Ward, W. E., Lewis, J. E., Hilditch, J., Nickell, L., Wong, E., and Thompson, L. U. 2004. Supplementation with flaxseed alters estrogen metabolism in postmenopausal women to a greater extent than does supplementation with an equal amount of soy. *American Journal of Clinical Nutrition* 79:318–325.

Brown, D. E. 1981. General stress in anthropological fieldwork. *American Anthropologist* 81:74–92.

Brown, D. E., James, G. D., Aki, S. L., Mills, P. S., and Etrata, M. B. 2003. A comparison of awake–sleep blood pressure variation between normotensive Japanese-American and Caucasian Women in Hawaii. *Journal of Hypertension* 21(11):2045–2051.

Brown, D. E., James, G. D., and Nordloh, L. 1998. Comparison of factors affecting daily variation of blood pressure in Filipino-American and Caucasian nurses in Hawaii. *American Journal of Physical Anthropology* 106(3):373–383.

Brown, D. E., Sievert, L. L., Aki, S. L., Mills, P. S., Etrata, M. B., Paopao, R.N.K., and James, G. D. 2001. The effects of age, ethnicity, and menopause on ambulatory blood pressure: Japanese-American and Caucasian school teachers in Hawaii. *American Journal of Human Biology* 13:486–493.

Brown, J. 1982. A cross-cultural exploration of the end of the childbearing years. In A. Voda, M. Dinnerstein, and S. O'Donnell, eds., *Changing Perspectives on Menopause*, 51–59. Austin: University of Texas Press.

Brown, P. J., and Konnor, M. 1987. An anthropological perspective on obesity. *Annals of the New York Academy of Sciences* 499:29–46.

Browner, C. H., Ortiz de Montellano, B.R.O., and Rubel, A. J. 1988. A methodology for cross-cultural ethnomedical research. *Current Anthropology* 29(5):681–689.

Buckley, T., and Gottlieb, A. 1988. A critical appraisal of theories of menstrual symbolism. In T. Buckley, and A. Gottlieb, eds., *Blood Magic: The Anthropology of Menstruation*, 3–50. Berkeley: University of California Press.

Buehler, J. W., Kaunitz, A. M., Hogue, C. J., Hughes, J. M., Smith, J. C., and Rochat, R. W. 1986. Maternal mortality in women aged 35 years or older: United States. *Journal of the American Medical Association* 255(1):53–57.

Bulbrook, R. D. 1991. Hormones and breast cancer. *Oxford Review of Reproductive Biology* 13:175–202.

Burger, H. G., Cahir, N., Robertson, D. M., Groome, N. P., Dudley, E., Green, A., and Dennerstein, L. 1998. Serum inhibins A and B fall differentially as FSH rises in perimenopausal women. *Clinical Endocrinology* 48:809–813.

Burger, H. G., Dudley, E. C., Hopper, J. L., Groome, N., Guthrie, J. R., Green, A., and Dennerstein, L. 1999. Prospectively measured levels of serum follicle stimulating hormone, estradiol, and the dimeric inhibins during the menopausal transition in a population-based cohort of women. *Journal of Clinical Endocrinology and Metabolism* 84:4025–4030.

Burger, H. G., Dudley, E. C., Hopper, J. L., Shelley, J. M., Greene, A., Smith, A., Dennerstein, L., and Morse, C. 1995. The endocrinology of the menopausal transition: a cross-sectional study of a population-based sample. *Journal of Clinical Endocrinology and Metabolism* 80:3537–3545.

Burger, H. G., Dudley, E., Mamers, P., Robertson, D., Groome, N., and Dennerstein, L. 2002. *The Ageing Female Reproductive Axis. I. Endocrine Facets of Ageing*, 161–171. Novartis Foundation Symposium 242. Chichester: Wiley.

Bustillo, M., Buster, J. E., Freeman, A. G., Gornbein, J. A., Wheeler, N., and Marshall, J. R. 1984. Nonsurgical ovum transfer as a treatment for intractable infertility: what effectiveness can we realistically expect? *American Journal of Obstetrics and Gynecology* 149(4):371–375.

Byskov, A. G. 1978. Follicular atresia. In R. E. Jones, ed., *The Vertebrate Ovary*, 533–562. New York: Plenum.

Cameron, N., and Demerath, E. W. 2002. Critical periods in human growth and their relationship to diseases of aging. *Yearbook of Physical Anthropology* 45:159–184.

Campagnoli, C., Morra, G., Belforte, P., Belforte, L., and Prelato Tousijn, L. 1981. Climacteric symptoms according to body weight in women of different socio-economic groups. *Maturitas* 3:279–287.

Candy, C. J., Wood, M. J., and Whittingham, D. G. 2000. Restoration of a normal reproductive lifespan after grafting of cryopreserved mouse ovaries. *Human Reproduction.* 15(6):1300–1304.

Canto-de-Cetina, T. E., Canto-Cetina, P., and Polanco-Reyes, L. 1998. Encuesta de síntomas del climaterio en áreas semirurales de Yucatán. *Revista de Investigación Clínica* 50:133–135.

Carda, S. N., Bilge, S. A., Ozturk, T. N., Oya, G., Ece, O., and Hamiyet, B. 1998. The menopausal age, related factors, and climacteric symptoms in Turkish women. *Maturitas* 30:37–40.

Carlisle, D. M., Valdez, R. B., Shapiro, M. F., and Brook, R. H. 1995. Geographic variation in rates of selected surgical procedures within Los Angeles County. *Health Services Research* 30:27–42.

Caro, T. M., Sellen, D. W., Parish, A., Frank, R., Brown, D. M., Voland, E., and Mulder, M. B. 1995. Termination of reproduction in nonhuman and human female primates. *International Journal of Primatology* 16(2):205–220.

Carpenter, J. S., Andrykowski, M. A., Cordova, M., Cunningham, L., Studts, J., McGrath, P., Kenady, D., Sloan, D., and Munn, R. 1998. Hot flashes in postmenopausal women treated for breast carcinoma: prevalence, severity, correlates, management, and relation to quality of life. *Cancer* 82(9):1682–1691.

Carpenter, J. S., Andrykowski, M. A., Freedman, R. R., and Munn, R. 1999. Feasibility and psychometrics of an ambulatory hot flash monitoring device. *Menopause* 6(3):209–215.

Carpenter, J. S., Gautam, S., Freedman, R. R., and Andrykowski, M. 2001. Circadian rhythm of objectively recorded hot flashes in postmenopausal breast cancer survivors. *Menopause* 8(3):181–188.

Carpenter, J. S., Gilchrist, J. M., Chen, K., Gautam, S., and Freedman, R. R. 2004. Hot flashes, core body temperature, and metabolic parameters in breast cancer survivors. *Menopause* 11(4):375–381.

Carpenter, J. S., Johnson, D. H., Wagner, L. J., and Andrykowsi, M. A. 2002. Hot flashes and related outcomes in breast cancer survivors and matched comparison women. *Oncology Nursing Forum* 29(3):E16–E25.

Cartwright, L. K. 1987. Role montage: life patterns of professional women. *Journal of the American Medical Women's Association* 42(5):142–148.

Caspari, R., and Lee, S. H. 2004. Older age becomes common late in human evolution. *Proceedings of the National Academy of Science* 101(30):10895–10900.

Casper, R. F., Graves, G. R., and Reid, R. L. 1987. Objective measurement of hot flushes associated with the premenstrual syndrome. *Fertility and Sterility* 47(2):341–344.

Casper, R. F., Yen, S.S.C., and Wilkes, M. M. 1979. Menopausal flushes: a neuroendocrine link with pulsatile luteinizing hormone secretion. *Science* 205:823–825.

Cattanach, J. 1985. Oestrogen deficiency after tubal ligation. *Lancet* 1(8433):847–849.

Cavalli-Sforza, L. L. 1983. The transition to agriculture and some of its consequences. In D. J. Ortner, ed., *How Humans Adapt: A Biocultural Odyssey*, 103–126. Washington, DC: Smithsonian Institute Press.

Center for Disease Control (CDC). 2001. *Women and smoking: a report of the Surgeon General— 2001.* www.cdc.gov/tobacco/sg_women.htm.

Chaikittisilpa, S., Chompootweep, S., Limpaphayom, K., and Taechakraichana, N. 1997. Symptoms and problems of menopausal women in Klong Toey slum. *Journal of the Medical Association of Thailand* 80:257–261.

Chandra, A. 1998. Surgical sterilization in the United States: prevalence and characteristics, 1965–1995. *Vital and Health Statistics.* Series 23 June (20):1–33.

Channing, C. P., Gordon, W. L., Liu, W. K., and Ward, D. N. 1985. Physiology and biochemistry of ovarian inhibin. *Proceedings of the Society for Experimental Biology and Medicine* 178:339–361.

Cheng, T. O. 2003. Lower body mass index cut-off values for obesity in China [letter]. *Nutrition Reviews* 61(12):432–433.

Chernyshov, V. P., Radysh, T. V., Gura, I. V., Tatarchuk, T. P., and Khominskaya, Z. B. 2001. Immune disorders in women with premature ovarian failure in initial period. *American Journal of Reproductive Immunology* 46(3):220–225.

Chetkowski, R. J., Rode, R. A., Burruel, V., and Nass, T. E. 1991. The effect of pituitary suppression and the women's age on embryo viability and uterine receptivity. *Fertility and Sterility* 56(6):1095–1103.

Chiechi, L. M., Ferreri, R., Granieri, M., Bianco, G., Berardesca, C., and Loizzi, P. 1997. Climacteric syndrome and body weight. *Clinical and Experimental Obstetrics and Gynecology* 24:163–166.

Cnattingius, S., Forman, M. R., Berendes, H. W., and Isotalo, L. 1992. Delayed childbearing and risk of adverse perinatal outcome: a population-based study. *Journal of the American Medical Association* 268(7):886–890.

Cohen, Y. A. 1952. A study of interpersonal relations in a Jamaican community. Ph.D. diss., Yale University.

Colditz, G. A., Stampfer, M. J., Willett, W. C., Stason, W. B., Rosner, B., Hennekens, C. H., and Speizer, F. E. 1987. Reproducibility and validity of self-reported menopausal status in a prospective cohort study. *American Journal of Epidemiology* 126:319–325.

Collaborative Group on Hormonal Factors in Breast Cancer. 1997. Breast cancer and hormone replacement therapy: collaborative reanalysis of data from 51 epidemiologic studies of 52,705 women with breast cancer and 108,411 women without breast cancer. *Lancet* 350:1047–1059.

Collins, A., and Landgren, B.-M. 1994. Experience of symptoms during transition to menopause: a population-based longitudinal study. In G. Berg, and M. Hammar, eds., *The Modern Management of the Menopause*, 71–77. New York: Parthenon Publishing.

Comfort, A. 1979. *The Biology of Scenescence*. Edinburgh: Churchill Livingstone.

Conrad, P. 1992. Medicalization and social control. *Annual Review of Sociology* 18:209–232.

Cooper, W. 1975. *Don't Change: A Biological Revolution for Women*. New York: Stein and Day.

Corson, S. L., Gutmann, J., Batzer, F. R., Wallace, H., Klein, N., and Soules, M. R. 1999. Inhibin-B as a test of ovarian reserve for infertile women. *Human Reproduction* 14(11):2818–2821.

Costoff, A., and Mahesh, V.B. 1975. Primordial follicles with normal oocytes in the ovaries of postmenopausal women. *Journal of the American Geriatrics Society* 23:193–196.

Coulam, C. B., Stringfellow, S., and Hoefnagel, D. 1983. Evidence for a genetic factor in the etiology of premature ovarian failure. *Fertility and Sterility* 40(5):693–695.

Coulter, A., McPherson, K., and Vessey, M. 1988. Do British women undergo too many or too few hysterectomies? *Social Science and Medicine* 27:987–994.

Cramer, D. W., Welch, W. R., Cassells, S., and Scully, R. E. 1983. Mumps, menarche, menopause, and ovarian cancer. *American Journal of Obstetrics and Gynecology* 147:1–6.

Cramer, D. W., Harlow, B. L., Barbieri, R., and Ng, W. G. 1989. Galactose-1-phosphate uridyl transferase activity associated with age at menopause and reproductive history. *Fertility and Sterility* 51:609–615.

Cramer, D. W., and Xu, H. 1996. Predicting age at menopause. *Maturitas* 23:319–326.

Cramer, D. W., Xu, H., and Harlow, B. L. 1995. Family history as a predictor of early menopause. *Fertility and Sterility* 64:740–745.

Cresswell, J. L., Egger, P., Fall, C. H., Osmond, C., Fraser, R. B., and Barker, D. J. 1997. Is the age of menopause determined in-utero? *Early Human Development* 49:143–148.

Crisp, T. M. 1992. Organization of the ovarian follicle and events in its biology: oogenesis, ovulation, or atresia. *Mutation Research* 296:89–106.

Csordas, T. J. 1994. *Embodiment and Experience: The Existentialist Ground of Culture*. New York: Cambridge University Press.

Currier, A. F. 1897. *The Menopause: A Consideration of the Phenomena Which Occur to Women at the Close of the Child-Bearing Period, with Incidental Allusions to Their Relationship to Menstruation. Also a Particular Consideration of the Premature (Especially the Artificial) Menopause*. New York: D. Appleton and Company.

Cutler, R. G. 1976. Evolution of longevity in primates. *Journal of Human Evolution* 5:169–202.

———. 1978. Alterations with age in the informational storage and flow systems of the mammalian cell. In D. Bergsma, and D. Harrison, eds., *Genetic Effects on Aging*, 463–498. New York: Alan R. Liss.

Cutler, W. B., and Garcia, C. R. 1984. *The Medical Management of the Menopause and Premenopause: Their Endocrinologic Basis*. Philadelphia: Lippincott Co.

Cutler, W. B., Preti, G., Krieger, A., Huggins, G. R., Garcia, C. R., and Lawley, H. J. 1986. Human axillary secretions influence women's menstrual cycles: the role of donor extract from men. *Hormones and Behavior* 20:463–473.

Daly, E., Vessey, M. P., Barlow, D., Gray, A., McPherson, K., and Roche, M. 1994. Hormone replacement therapy in a risk–benefit perspective. In G. Berg, and M. Hammar, eds., *The Modern Management of the Menopause: A Perspective for the Twenty First Century*, 473–497. New York: Parthenon Publishing Group.

Damewood, M. D., Zacur, H. A., Hoffman, G. J., and Rock, J. A. 1986. Circulating antiovarian antibodies in premature ovarian failure. *Obstetrics and Gynecology* 68(6):850–854.

Danforth, D. R., Arbogast, L. K., Mroueh, J., Kim, M. H., Kennard, E. A., Seifer, D. B., and Friedman, C. I. 1998. Dimeric inhibin: a direct marker of ovarian aging. *Fertility and Sterility* 70(1):119–123.

Datan, N., Antonovsky, A., and Maoz, B. 1981. *A Time to Reap: The Middle Age of Women in Five Israeli Subcultures*. Baltimore: Johns Hopkins University Press.

Davenport, F. H. 1898. *Diseases of Women: A Manual of Gynecology Designed Especially for the Use of Students and General Practitioners*. Philadelphia: Lea Brothers and Co.

Davis, D. L. 1983. *Blood and Nerves: An Ethnographic Focus on Menopause*. Social and Economic Studies no. 28, St. John's, Newfoundland: Institute of Social and Economic Research, Memorial University of Newfoundland.

———. 1986. The meaning of menopause in a Newfoundland fishing village. *Culture, Medicine, and Psychiatry* 10:73–94.

Dawkins, R. 1976. *The Selfish Gene*. New York: Oxford University Press.

de Bakker, I.P.M., and Everaerd, W. 1996. Measurement of menopausal hot flushes: validation and cross-validation. *Maturitas* 25:87–98.

de Bruin, J. P., Bovenhuis, H., van Noord, P.A.H., Pearson, P. L., van Arendonk, J.A.M., te Velde, E. R., Kuurman, W. W., and Dorland, M. 2001. The role of genetic factors in age at natural menopause. *Human Reproduction* 16(9):2014–2018.

Delaney, J., Lupton, M. J., and Toth, E. 1988. *The Curse: A Cultural History of Menstruation*. Chicago: University of Illinois Press.

Dennerstein, L. 1994. In pursuit of happiness: well-being during the menopausal transition. In G. Berg, and M. Hammar, eds., *The Modern Management of the Menopause: A Perspective for the Twenty First Century*, 151–159. New York: Parthenon Publishing Group.

———. 1996. Well-being, symptoms, and the menopausal transition. *Maturitas* 23:147–157.

Dennerstein, L., Dudley, E. C., Hopper, J. L., Guthrie, J. R., and Burger, H. G. 2000. A prospective population-based study of menopausal symptoms. *Obstetrics and Gynecology* 96:351–358.

Dennerstein, L., Smith, A.M.A., Morse, C., Burger, H., Green, A., Hopper, J., and Ryan, M. 1993. Menopausal symptoms in Australian women. *Medical Journal of Australia* 159:232–236.

den Tonkelaar, I., Broekmans, F. J., de Boer, E. J., te Velde, E. R. 2002. Letter to the editor. *Menopause* 9(6):463–464.

den Tonkelaar, I., Seidell, J. C., and van Noord, P.A.H. 1996. Obesity and fat distribution in relation to hot flashes in Dutch women from the DOM-project. *Maturitas* 23:301–305.

Dettwyler, K. 1995a. A time to wean: the hominid blueprint for the natural age of weaning in modern human populations. In P. Stuart-Macadam, and K. A. Dettwyler, eds., *Breastfeeding: Biocultural Perspectives*, 39–73. Hawthorne, NY: Aldine de Gruyter.

———. 1995b. Beauty and the breast: the cultural context of breastfeeding in the United States. In P. Stuart-Macadam, and K. A. Dettwyler, eds., *Breastfeeding: Biocultural Perspectives*, 167–215. Hawthorne, NY: Aldine de Gruyter.

Deurenberg-Yap, M., and Deurenberg, P. 2003. Is a re-evaluation of WHO body mass index cut-off values needed? The case of Asians in Singapore. *Nutrition Reviews* 61:S80–S87.

de Vet, A., Laven, J. S., de Jong, F. H., Themmen, A. P., and Fauser, B. C. 2002. Antimüllerian hormone serum levels: a putative marker for ovarian aging. *Fertility and Sterility* 77(2):357–362.

De Young, J. E. 1955. *Village Life in Modern Thailand.* Berkeley: University of California Press.

Diagnostic and Statistics Manual–II (DSM-II). 1968. *Diagnostic and Statistical Manual of Mental Disorders.* 2nd ed. Washington, DC: American Psychiatric Association.

Dickinson, F., Castillo, T., Vales, L., and Uc, L. 1992. Migration, socio-economic status, and age at menarche and age at menopause in the Yucatan, Mexico. *International Journal of Anthropology* 10:21–28.

Do, K.-A., Treloar, S. A., Pandeya, N., Purdie, D., Green, A. C., Heath, A. C., and Martin, N. G. 1998. Predictive factors of age at menopause in a large Australian twin study. *Human Biology* 70(6):1073–1091.

Dobson, H., Ghuman, S., Prabhaker, S., and Smith, R. 2003. A conceptual model of the influence of stress on female reproduction. *Reproduction* 125(2):151–163.

Donaldson, J. F. 1984. Did the experience of the African savanna bring about the human menopause? *Central African Journal of Medicine* 30:198–201.

———. 1994. How did the human menopause arise? *Menopause* 1:211–221.

Donnez, J., Dolmans, M. M., Demylle, D., Jadoul, P., Pirard, C., Squifflet, J., Martinez-Madrid, B., and van Langendonckt, A. 2004. Livebirth after orthotopic transplantation of cryopreserved ovarian tissue. *Lancet* 364(9443):1405–1410.

Dressler, W. W. 1995. Modeling biocultural interactions in anthropological research: an example from research on stress and cardiovascular disease. *Yearbook of Physical Anthropology* 38:27–56.

———. 1996. Culture, stress, and disease. In T. M. Johnson, and C. F. Sargent, eds., *Medical Anthropology: Contemporary Theory and Method,* 252–271. Westport, CT: Praeger.

Dressler, W. W., and Bindon, J. R. 2000. The health consequences of cultural consonance: cultural dimensions of lifestyle, social support, and arterial blood pressure in an African American community. *American Anthropologist* 102:244–260.

Durham, W. H. 1991. *Coevolution: Genes, Culture and Human Diversity.* Stanford, CA: Stanford University Press.

Dyke, B., Gage, T. B., Mamelka, P. M., Goy, R. W., and Stone, W. H. 1986. A demographic analysis of the Wisconsin Regional Primate Center Rhesus colony, 1962–1982. *American Journal of Primatology* 10(3):257–269.

Eaton, S. B., and Eaton, S. B. 1999. Breast cancer in evolutionary context. In W. Trevathan, E. O. Smith, and J. J. McKenna, eds., *Evolutionary Medicine,* 429–442. New York: Oxford University Press.

Eaton, S. B., Eaton S. B., and Konner, M. J. 1999. Paleolithic nutrition revisited. In W. R. Trevathan, E. O. Smith, and J. J. McKenna, eds., *Evolutionary Medicine,* 313–332. New York: Oxford University Press.

Eaton, S. B., Pike, M. C., Short, R. V., Lee, N. C., Trussell, J., Hatcher, R. A., Wood, J. W., Worthman, C. M., Jones, N.G.B., Konner, M. J., Hill, K. R., Bailey, R., and Hurtado, A. M. 1994. Women's reproductive cancers in evolutionary context. *Quarterly Review of Biology* 69:353–366.

Edgewater, I. D. 1999. Music hath charms . . . fragments toward constructionist biocultural theory, with attention to the relationship of "music" and "emotion." In A. L. Hinton, ed., *Biocultural Approaches to the Emotions*, 153–181. Cambridge: Cambridge University Press.

Edwards, R. G. 1993. Pregnancies are acceptable in post-menopausal women. *Human Reproduction* 8:1542–1544.

Einspanier, A., and Gore, M. A. 2005. Reproduction: definition of a primate model of female fertility. In S. Wolfe-Coote, ed., *The Laboratory Primate*, 105–117. Boston: Elsevier Academic Press.

Elder, G. H. 1985. Perspective on the life course. In G. H. Elder, ed., *Life Course Dynamics: Trajectories and Transitions, 1968–1980*, 23–49. Ithaca, NY: Cornell University Press.

Elias, S. G., van Noord, P. A., Peeters, P. H., den Tonkelaar, I., and Grobbee, D. E. 2003. Caloric restriction reduces age at menopause: the effect of the 1944–1945 Dutch famine. *Menopause* 10(5):399–405.

Elinson, L., Cohen, M. M., and Elmslie, T. 1999. Hormone replacement therapy: a survey of Ontario physicians' prescribing practices. *Canadian Medical Association Journal* 161(6):695–698.

Elkind-Hirsch, K. 2004. Cooling off hot flashes: uncoupling of the circadian pattern of core body temperature and hot flash frequency in breast cancer survivors. *Menopause* 11(4):369–371.

Ellison, P. T. 1999. Reproductive ecology and reproductive cancers. In C. Panter-Brick, and C. M. Worthman, eds., *Hormones, Health, and Behavior*, 184–209. New York: Cambridge University Press.

———. 2001a. *On Fertile Ground*. Cambridge, MA: Harvard University Press.

———. 2001b. *Reproductive Ecology and Human Evolution*. New York: Aldine de Gruyter.

Emmens, D. J. 1998. The experience of menopause for fifty Auckland women and its relation to reproductive life history. MA thesis, Department of Anthropology, University of Auckland.

Enmark, E., Pelto-Huikko, M., Grandien, K., Lagercrantz, S., Lagercrantz, J., Fried, G., Nordenskjold, M., and Gustafsson, J. A. 1997. Human estrogen receptor beta-gene structure, chromosomal localization, and expression pattern. *Journal of Clinical Endocrinology and Metabolism* 82(12):4258–4265.

Erickson, G. F. 2000. Ovarian anatomy and physiology. In R. A. Lobo, J. Kelsey, and R. Marcus, eds., *Menopause: Biology and Pathobiology*, 13–31. New York: Academic Press.

Erlik, Y., Meldrum, D. R., Judd, H. L. 1982. Estrogen levels in postmenopausal women with hot flashes. *Obstetrics and Gynecology* 59:403–407.

Ettinger, B., and Grady, D. 1993. The waning effect of postmenopausal estrogen therapy on osteoporosis. *New England Journal of Medicine* 329(16):1192–1193.

Evans, J. G. 1981. The biology of human ageing. *Recent Advances in Medicine* 18:17–38.

Eveleth, P. B., and Tanner, J. M. 1990. *Worldwide Variation in Human Growth*. 2nd ed. New York: Cambridge University Press.

Faddy, M. J., Gosden, R. G., Gougeon, A., Richardson, S. J., and Nelson, J. F. 1992. Accelerated disappearance of ovarian follicles in mid-life: implications for forecasting menopause. *Human Reproduction* 7:1342–1346.

Falk, D. 1992. *Brain Dance: New Discoveries about Human Origins and Brain Evolution*. New York: Henry Holt and Company.

Familiari, G., Caggiati, A., Nottola, S. A., Ermini, M., DiBenedetto, M. R., and Motta, P. M. 1993. Ultrastructure of human ovarian primordial follicles after combination chemotherapy for Hodgkin's disease. *Human Reproduction* 8(12):2080–2087.

Farquhar, C. M., and Steiner, C. A. 2002. Hysterectomy rates in the United States, 1990–1997. *Obstetrics and Gynecology* 99:229–234.

Federation CECOS, Schwartz, D., and Mayaux, M. J. 1982. Female fecundity as a function of age: results of artificial insemination in 2193 nulliparous women with azoospermic husbands. *New England Journal of Medicine* 306(7):404–406.

Feldman, B. M., Voda, A., and Gronseth, E. 1985. The prevalence of hot flash and associated variables among perimenopausal women. *Research in Nursing and Health* 8:261–268.

Felson, D. T., and Nevitt, M. C. 1999. Estrogen and osteoarthritis: how do we explain conflicting study results? *Preventive Medicine* 28:445–448.

Ferin, M., Van Vugt, D., and Wardlaw, S. 1984. The hypothalamic control of the menstrual cycle and the role of the endogenous opioid peptides. *Recent Progress in Hormonal Research* 40:441–485.

Field, M. J. 1962. *Search for Security: An Ethno-Psychiatric Study of Rural Ghana*. Evanston, IL: Northwestern University Press.

Filipp, S.-H., and Olbrich, E. 1986. Human development across the life span: overview and highlights of the psychological perspective. In A. G. Sorensen, F. E. Weinert, and L. R. Sherrod, eds., *Human Development and the Life Course: Multidisciplinary Perspectives*, 343–375. Hillsdale, NJ: Lawrence Erlbaum Associates.

Finch, C. E. 1990. *Longevity, Senescence, and the Genome*. Chicago: University of Chicago Press.

Finch, C. E, and Gosden, R. 1986. Animal models for the human menopause. In L. Mastroianni, and C. A. Paulsen, eds., *Aging, Reproduction, and the Climacteric*, 3–34. New York: Plenum.

Finkler, K. 1994. *Women in Pain: Gender and Morbidity in Mexico*. Philadelphia: University of Pennsylvania Press.

Finney, D. J. 1962. *Probit Analysis: Statistical Treatment of the Sigmoid Response Curve*. Cambridge: Cambridge University Press.

Fisher, S. 1986. *In the Patient's Best Interest: Women and the Politics of Medical Decisions*. New Brunswick, NJ: Rutgers University Press.

Fitch, N., de Saint Victor, J., Richer, L. C., Pinsky, L., and Sitahal, S. 1982. Premature menopause due to a small deletion in the long arm of the X chromosome; a report of 3 cases and a review. *American Journal of Obstetrics and Gynecology* 142:968–972.

Flaws, J. A., Langenberg, P., Babus, J. K., Hirshfield, A. N., and Sharara, F. I. 2001. Ovarian volume and antral follicle counts as indictors of menopausal status. *Menopause* 8:175–180.

Flaws, J. A., Rhodes, J. C., Langenberg, P., Hirshfeld, A. N., Kjerulff, K., and Sharara, F. I. 2000. Ovarian volume and menopause status. *Menopause* 7:53–61.

Flaxman, S. M., and Sherman, P. W. 2000. Morning sickness: a mechanism for protecting mother and embryo. *Quarterly Review of Biology* 75(2):113–148.

Flint, M. 1974. Menarche and menopause of Rajput women. Ph.D. diss., City University of New York.

———. 1975. The menopause: reward or punishment? *Psychosomatics*. 16:161–163.

———. 1997. Secular trends in menopause age. *Journal of Psychosomatic Obstetrics and Gynaecology* 18:65–72.

Flint, M., and Garcia, M. 1979. Culture and the climacteric. *Journal of Biosocial Science* (supp.)6:197–215.

Flint, M., and Samil, R. 1990. Cultural and subcultural meanings of the menopause. *Annals of the New York Academy of Sciences* 592:134–138.

Forbes, L. S. 1997. The evolutionary biology of spontaneous abortion in humans. *Trends in Ecology and Evolution* 12:446–450.

Ford, G. 1993. *What's Wrong with My Hormones?* Rocklin, CA: J & M Printing.

Ford, H. 1975. Involutional melancholia. In A. M. Freedman, H. I. Kaplan, and B. J. Sadock, eds., *Comprehensive Textbook of Psychiatry II.* 2nd ed., 1025–1042. Baltimore: Williams and Wilkins Co.

Foster, P. 1995. *Women and the Health Care Industry: An Unhealthy Relationship?* Philadelphia: Open University Press.

Freedman, R. R. 1989. Laboratory and ambulatory monitoring of menopausal hot flashes. *Psychophysiology* 26:573–579.

———. 1998. Biochemical, metabolic, and vascular mechanisms in menopausal hot flashes. *Fertility and Sterility* 70:332–337.

———. 2000a. Menopausal hot flashes. In R. A. Lobo, J. Kelsey, and R. Marcus, eds., *Menopause: Biology and Pathology,* 215–227. New York: Academic Press.

———. 2000b. Hot flashes revisited [editorial]. *Menopause* 7:3–4.

———. 2002. Hot flash trends and mechanisms *Menopause* 9:151–152.

Freedman, R. R., and Blacker, C.M.S.O. 2002. Estrogen raises the sweating threshold in post-menopausal women with hot flashes. *Fertility and Sterility* 77(3):487–490.

Freedman, R. R., and Dinsay, R. 2000. Clonidine raises the sweating threshold in symptomatic but not in asymptomatic postmenopausal women. *Fertility and Sterility* 74:20–23.

Freedman, R. R., and Krell, W. 1999. Reduced thermoregulatory null zone in post-menopausal women with hot flashes. *American Journal of Obstetrics and Gynecology* 181:66–70.

Freedman, R. R., Norton, D., Woodward, S., and Cornelissen, G. 1995. Core body temperature and circadian rhythm of hot flashes in menopausal women. *Journal of Clinical Endocrinology and Metabolism* 80(8):2354–2358.

Freedman, R. R., and Woodward, S. 1992. Elevated alpha-2 adrenergic responsiveness in menopausal hot flushes: pharmacologic and biochemical studies. In P. Lomax and E. Schonbaum, eds., *Thermoregulation: The Pathophysiological Basis of Clinical Disorders,* 6–9. Basel: Karger.

———. 1996. Core body temperature during menopausal hot flushes. *Fertility and Sterility* 65(6):1141–1144.

Freedman, R. R., Woodward, S., and Norton, D.A.M. 1992. Laboratory and ambulatory monitoring of menopausal hot flushes: comparison of symptomatic and asymptomatic women. *Journal of Psychophysiology* 6:162–166.

Freeman, E. W., Sammel, M. D., Grisso, J. A., Battistini, M., Garcia-Espagna, B., and Hollander, L. 2001. Hot flashes in the late reproductive years: risk factors for African American and Caucasian women. *Journal of Women's Health* 10(1):67–76.

Fretts, R. C., Schmittdiel, J., McLean, F. H., Usher, R. H., and Goldman, M. B. 1995. Increased maternal age and the risk of fetal death. *New England Journal of Medicine* 333:953–957.

Friede, A., Baldwin, W., Rhodes, P. H., Buehler, J. W., Strauss, L. T. 1988. Older maternal age and infant mortality in the United States. *Obstetrics and Gynecology* 72(2):152–157.

Frisancho, A. R. 1993. *Human Adaptation and Accommodation*. Ann Arbor: University of Michigan Press.

Frisch, R. E. 1978. Population, food intake, and fertility. *Science* 199:22–29.

Fuleihan, G.E.-H. 1997. Tissue-specific estrogens—the promise for the future [editorial]. *New England Journal of Medicine* 337:1686–1687.

Gage, T. B. 1998. The comparative demography of primates: with some comments on the evolution of life histories. *Annual Review of Anthropology* 27:197–221.

Gage, T. B., McCullough, J. M., Weitz, C. A., Dutt, J. S., and Abelson, A. 1989. Demographic studies and human population biology. In M. A. Little, and J. D. Haas, eds., *Human Population Biology: A Transdisciplinary Science*, 45–65. New York: Oxford University Press.

Gannon, L., Ekstrom, B. 1993. Attitudes toward menopause: the influence of sociocultural paradigms. *Psychology of Women Quarterly* 17:275–288.

García Vela, A., Nava, L. E., and Malacara, J. M. 1987. La edad de la menopausia en la población urbana de la ciudad de León, Gto. *La Revista de Investigación Clínica* (Mexico) 39:329–332.

Garrido-Latorre, F., Lazcano-Ponce, E. C., López-Carrillo, L., and Hernández-Avila, M. 1996. Age of natural menopause among women in Mexico City. *International Journal of Gynecology and Obstetrics* 53:159–166.

Gath, D., and Isles, S. 1990. Depression and the menopause. *British Medical Journal* 300:1287–1288.

Gaulin, S.J.C. 1980. Sexual dimorphism in the human post-reproductive life-span: possible causes. *Journal of Human Evolution* 9:227–232.

Gavaler, J. S. 1985. A review of alcohol effects on endocrine function in postmenopausal women: what we know, what we need to know, and what we do not yet know. *Journal of Studies on Alcohol* 46:495–516.

Geller, S. E., Burns, L. R., and Brailer, D. J. 1996. The impact of nonclinical factors on practice variations: the case of hysterectomies. *Health Services Research* 30:729–750.

Genazzani, A. D., Petraglia, F., Sgarbi, L., Montanini, V., Hartmann, B., Surico, N., Biolcati, A., Volpe, A., and Genazzani, A. R. 1997. Difference of LH and FSH secretory characteristics and degree of concordance between postmenopausal and aging women. *Maturitas* 26:133–138.

Genazzani, A. R., Bernardi, F., Monteleone, P., Luisi, S., and Luisi, M. 2000. Neuropeptides, neurotransmitters, neurosteroids, and the onset of puberty. *Annals of the New York Academy of Sciences* 900:1–9.

Gentile, G. P., Kaufman, S. C., and Helbig, D. W. 1998. Is there any evidence for a post-tubal sterilization syndrome? *Fertility and Sterility* 69(2):179–186.

Gerber, L. M., Schwartz, J. E., Schnall, P. L., Devereux, R. B., Warren, K., and Pickering, T. G. 1999. Effect of body weight changes on changes in ambulatory and standardized non-physician blood pressures over three years. *Annals of Epidemiology* 9(8):489–497.

Gibson, M. A., and Mace, R. 2002. Labor-saving technology and fertility increase in rural Africa. *Current Anthropology* 43(4):631–637.

Gill, J. 2000. The effects of moderate alcohol consumption on female hormone levels and reproductive function. *Alcohol and Alcoholism* 35(5):417–423.

Ginsburg, J., and O'Reilly, B. 1983. Climacteric flushing in a man. *British Medical Journal* 287(6387):262.

Gladwin, T., and Sarason, S. S. 1953. *Truk: Man in Paradise*. Viking Fund Publication in Anthropology no. 20. New York: Wenner-Gren Foundation.

Gold, E. B., Sternfeld, B., Kelsey, J. L., Brown, C., Mouton, C., Reame, N., Salamone, L., and Stellato, R. 2000. Relation of demographic and lifestyle factors to symptoms in a multi-racial/ethnic population of women 40–55 years of age. *American Journal of Epidemiology* 152(5):463–473.

Goldhaber, M. K., Armstrong, M. A., Golditch, I. M., Sheehe, P. R., Petitti, D. B., and Friedman, G. D. 1993. Long-term risk of hysterectomy among 80,007 sterilized and comparison women at Kaiser Permanente, 1971–1987. *American Journal of Epidemiology* 138(7):508–521.

Gonzales, G. F., and Villena, A. 1997. Age at menopause in central Andean Peruvian women. *Menopause* 4(1):32–38.

González Quintero, L., and López Alonso, S. 2003. Vivir conviviendo: el nicho funcional, epítome de las estrategias de vida y de reproducción en Atla, Puebla, México. *Estudios de Antropología Biológica* 11:139–154.

Goodall, J. 1990. *Through a Window: My Thirty Years with the Chimpanzees of Gombe*. Boston: Houghton Mifflin.

Goodfriend, J. D., and Christie, C. M. 1988. *Lives of American Women: A History with Documents*. Lanham, MD: University Press of America.

Goodman, A., and Leatherman, T. 1998. *Building a New Biocultural Synthesis: Political-Economic Perspectives on Human Biology*. Ann Arbor: University of Michigan Press.

Goodman, M. 1980. Toward a biology of menopause. *Signs* 5:739–753.

Goodman, M., Estioko-Griffin, A., Griffin, P., and Grove, J. 1985. Menarche, pregnancy, birth spacing, and menopause among the Agta women foragers of Cagayan Province, Luzon, the Philippines. *Annals of Human Biology* 12:169–177.

Goodman, M. J., Stewart, C. J., and Gilbert, F. 1977. Patterns of menopause: a study of certain medical and physiological variables among Caucasian and Japanese women living in Hawaii. *Journal of Gerontology* 32(3):291–298.

Gordon, C. C., Chumlea, W. C., and Roche, A. F. 1988. Stature, recumbent length, and weight. In T. G. Lohman, A. F. Roche, and R. Martorell, eds., *Anthropometric Standardization Reference Manual*, 3–8. Champaign, IL: Human Kinetics Books.

Gosden, R. G. 1985. *Biology of Menopause: The Causes and Consequences of Ovarian Ageing*. New York: Academic Press.

Gosden, R. G., Baird, D. T., Wade, J. C., and Webb, R. 1994. Restoration of fertility to oophorectomized sheep by ovarian autografts stored at −196 degrees C. *Human Reproduction* 9(4):597–603.

Gosden, R. G., Wade, J. C., Fraser, H. M., Sandow, J., and Faddy, M. J. 1997. Impact of congenital or experimental hypogonadotrophism on the radiation sensitivity of the mouse ovary. *Human Reproduction* 12(11):2483–2488.

Gougeon, A. 1996. Regulation of ovarian follicular development in primates: facts and hypotheses. *Endocrine Reviews* 17:121–155.

Gougeon, A., Ecochard, R., and Thalabard, J. C. 1994. Age-related changes of the population of human ovarian follicles: increase in the disappearance rate of non-growing and early-growing follicles in aging women. *Biology of Reproduction* 50:653–663.

Gould, K. G., Flint, M., and Graham, C. E. 1981. Chimpanzee reproductive senescence: a possible model for evolution of the menopause. *Maturitas* 3:157–166.

Gould, S. J., and Lewontin, R. C. 1979. The spandrels of San Marco and the Panglossian paradigm: a critique of the adaptationist programme. *Proceedings of the Royal Society of London* B 205:581–598.

Grady, D., Herrington, D., Bittner, V., Blumenthal, R., Davidson, M., Hlatky, M., Hsia, J., Hulley, S., Herd, A., Khan, S., Newby, L. K., Waters, D., Vittinghoff, E., Wenger, N., and HERS Research Group. 2002. Cardiovascular disease outcomes during 6.8 years of hormone therapy: Heart and Estrogen/progestin Replacement Study follow-up (HERS II). *Journal of the American Medical Association* 288(1):49–57.

Graham, C. E. 1979. Reproductive function in aged female chimpanzees. *American Journal of Physical Anthropology* 50:291–300.

Granqvist, H. N. 1931. *Marriage Conditions in a Palestinian Village, I.* Commentationes Humanarum Litterarum, III(8). Helsingfors, Finland: Societas Scientiarum Fennica.

Granqvist, H. N. 1935. *Marriage Conditions in a Palestinian Village, II.* Commentationes Humanarum Litterarum, VI(8). Helsingfors, Finland: Societas Scientiarum Fennica.

Gray, R. H. 1976. The menopause—epidemiological and demographic considerations. In R. J. Beard, ed., *The Menopause: A Guide to Current Research and Practice,* 25–40. Baltimore: University Park Press.

Greene, J. G. 1976. A factor analytic study of climacteric symptoms. *Journal of Psychosomatic Research* 20(5):425–430.

———. 1998. Constructing a standard climacteric scale. *Maturitas* 29:25–31.

Greenspan, F. S., and Baxter, J. D. 1994. *Basic and Clinical Endocrinology.* 4th ed. Norwalk, CT: Appleton and Lange.

Griffiths, F. 1999. Women's control and choice regarding HRT. *Social Science and Medicine* 49(4):469–481.

Grisso, J. A., Freeman, E. W., Maurin, E., Garcia-Espana, B., and Berlin, J. A. 1999. Racial differences in menopause information and the experience of hot flashes. *Journal of General Internal Medicine* 14:98–103.

Guedes Pinto da Cunha, E. M. 1984. Estudo da idade da menopausa em Ançã e Coimbra: análise comparativa. *Antropologia Portuguesa* 2:9–19.

Guraya, S. S. 1985. *Biology of Ovarian Follicles in Mammals.* New York: Springer-Verlag.

Guthrie, J. R., Dennerstein, L., Hopper, J. L., and Burger, H. G. 1996. Hot flashes, menstrual status, and hormone levels in a population-based sample of midlife women. *Obstetrics and Gynecology* 88:437–442.

Haas, S., Acker, D., Donahue, C., and Katz, M. E. 1993. Variation in hysterectomy rates across small geographic areas of Massachusetts. *American Journal of Obstetrics and Gynecology* 169(1):150–154.

Hagestad, G. O. 1996. Thoughts about the life course. In D. A. Neugarten, ed., *The Meanings of Age: Selected Papers of Bernice L. Neugarten,* 81–87. Chicago: University of Chicago Press.

Hagstad, A., and Janson, P. O. 1986. The epidemiology of climacteric symptoms. *Acta Obstetricia et gynecologica Scandinavica* (supp.)134:59–65.

Hahn, P. M., Wong, J., and Reid, R. L. 1998. Menopausal-like hot flashes reported in women of reproductive age. *Fertility and Sterility* 70:913–918.

Hahn, R. A. 1995. *Sickness and Healing: An Anthropological Perspective.* New Haven, CT: Yale University Press.

Hahn, R. A., Eaker, E., and Rolka, H. 1997. Reliability of reported age at menopause. *American Journal of Epidemiology* 146:771–775.

Hall, R. 2004. An energetics-based approach to understanding the menstrual cycle and menopause. *Human Nature* 15(1):83–99.

Hall, R. E., and Cohen, M. M. 1994. Variations in hysterectomy rates in Ontario: does the indication matter? *Canadian Medical Association Journal* 151(12):1713–1719.

Hames, R. 1984. On the definition and measure of inclusive fitness and the evolution of menopause. *Human Ecology* 12:87–91.

Hamilton, W. D. 1966. The moulding of senescence by natural selection. *Journal of Theoretical Biology* 12:12–45.

Hammar, M., Berg, G., Fahraeus, L., and Larsson-Cohn, U. 1984. Climacteric symptoms in an unselected sample of Swedish women. *Maturitas* 6: 345–350.

Hardy, R., and Kuh, D. 2002a. Change in psychological and vasomotor symptom reporting during the menopause. *Social Science and Medicine* 55(11):1975–1988.

———. 2002b. Does early growth influence timing of the menopause? Evidence from a British birth cohort. *Human Reproduction* 17:2474–2479.

———. 2005. Social and environmental conditions across the life course and age at menopause in a British birth cohort study. *British Journal of Obstetrics and Gynecology* 112(3):346–354.

Harrel, B. B. 1977. Lactation and menstruation in cultural perspective. *American Anthropologist* 83:796–823.

Harris, C. 1987. The individual and society: a processual approach. In A. Bryman, B. Bythway, P. Allatt, and T. Keil, eds., *Rethinking the Life Cycle*, 17–29. London: Macmillan.

Hautaniemi, S. I., and Sievert, L. L. 2003. Risk factors for hysterectomy among Mexican American women in the U.S. Southwest. *American Journal of Human Biology* 15:38–47.

Hawkes, K., O'Connell, J. F., and Blurton Jones, N. G. 1997. Hadza women's time allocation, offspring provisioning and the evolution of post-menopausal lifespans. *Current Anthropology* 38:551–578.

———. 2001. Hadza meat sharing. *Evolution and Human Behavior* 22:113–142.

Hemminki, E., Topo, P., and Kangas, I. 1995. Experience and opinions of climacterium by Finnish women. *European Journal of Obstetrics and Gynecology* 62:81–87.

Hemminki, E., Topo, P., Malin, M., and Kangas, I. 1993. Physicians views on hormone therapy around and after menopause. *Maturitas* 16(3):163–173.

Henderson, B. E., Ross, R. K., Judd, H. L., Krailo, M. D., and Pike, M. C. 1985. Do regular ovulatory cycles increase breast cancer risk? *Cancer* 56:1206–1208.

Henderson, H. K. 1969. Ritual roles of women in Onitsha Igbo society. Ph.D. diss., University of California, Berkeley.

Herbison, A. E. 1997. Noradrenergic regulation of cyclic GnRH secretion. *Reviews of Reproduction* 2:1–6.

Hill, K., and Hurtado, A. M. 1991. The evolution of premature reproductive senescence and menopause in human females: an evaluation of the "grandmother hypothesis". *Human Nature* 2:313–350.

———. 1996. *Aché Life History: The Ecology and Demography of a Foraging People*. New York: Aldine de Gruyter.

Hill, J. O., Wyatt, H. R., Reed, G. W., and Peters, J. C. 2003. Obesity and the environment: where do we go from here? *Science* 299:853–855.

Hillis, S. D., Marchbanks, P. A., Tylor, L. R., and Peterson, H. B. 1998. Higher hysterectomy risk for sterilized than nonsterilized women: findings from the U.S. collaborative review of sterilization. *Obstetrics and Gynecology* 91:241–246.

Hinton, A. L. 1999. Introduction: developing a biocultural approach to the emotions. In A. L. Hinton, ed., *Biocultural Approaches to the Emotions*, 1–37. New York: Cambridge University Press.

Hodgen, G., Goodman, A., O'Connor, A., and Johnson, D. 1977. Menopause in rhesus monkeys: model for study of disorders in the human climacteric. *American Journal of Obstetrics and Gynecology* 127:581–584.

Holman, D. J., O'Connor, K. A., Brindle, E., Wood, J. W., Mansfield, P. K., and Weinstein, M. 2002. Ovarian follicular development in postmenopausal women [abstract]. *American Journal of Human Biology* 14(1):115.

Holman, D. J., Wood, J. W., and Campbell, K. L. 2000. Age-dependent decline of female fecundity is caused by early fetal loss. In E. R. te Velde, F. Broekmans, and P. Pearson, eds., *Female Reproductive Ageing*, 123–136. Studies in Profertiity Series 9. Camforth, UK: Parthenon.

Holte, A. 1991. Prevalence of climacteric complaints in a representative sample of middle-aged women in Oslo, Norway. *Journal of Psychosomatic Obstetrics and Gynaecology* 12:303–317.

———. 1992. Influences of natural menopause on health complaints: a prospective study of healthy Norwegian women. *Maturitas* 14:127–141.

Holte, A., and Mikkelsen, A. 1991a. Psychosocial determinants of climacteric complaints. *Maturitas* 13(3):205–215.

———. 1991b. The menopausal syndrome: a factor analytic replication. *Maturitas* 13(3):193–203.

Hrdy, S. B. 1999. *Mother Nature: A History of Mothers, Infants, and Natural Selection.* New York: Pantheon.

Huerta, R., Mena, A., Malacara, J. M., and Díaz de León, J. 1995. Symptoms at perimenopausal period: its association with attitudes toward sexuality, life-style, family function, and FSH levels. *Psychoneuroendocrinology* 20:135–148.

Huerta, R., Malacara, J. M., Fajardo, M. E., Nava, L. E., Bocanegra, A., and Sanchez, J. 1997. High-frequency FSH and LH pulses in obese menopausal women. *Endocrine* 7(3):281–286.

Huggins, G. R., and Sondheimer, S. J. 1984. Complications of female sterilization: immediate and delayed. *Fertility and Sterility* 41(3):337–355.

Hulley, S., Grady, D., Bush, T., Burberg, C., Herrington, D., Riggs, B., Vittinghoff, E. 1998. Randomized trial of estrogen plus progestin for secondary prevention of coronary heart disease in postmenopausal women. Heart and Estrogen/progestin Replacement Study (HERS) Research Group. *Journal of the American Medical Association* 280(7):605–613.

Hunter, M. S. 1990. Psychological and somatic experience of the menopause: a prospective study. *Psychosomatic Medicine* 52:357–367.

———. 1992. The South-East England longitudinal study of the climacteric and postmenopause. *Maturitas* 14:117–126.

———. 1993. Predictors of menopausal symptoms: psychosocial aspects. *Baillière's Clinical Endocrinology and Metabolism* 7:33–45.

———. 1994. The effects of estrogen therapy on mood and well-being. In G. Berg and M. Hammar, eds., *The Modern Management of the Menopause*, 177–184. New York: Parthenon Publishing.

Hunter, M., Battersby, R., and Whitehead, M. I. 1986. Relationships between psychological symptoms, somatic complaints, and menopausal status. *Maturitas* 8:217–228.

Hunter, R.H.F. 2003. *Physiology of the Graafian Follicle and Ovulation.* Cambridge: Cambridge University Press.

Indira, S. N., and Murthy V. N. 1980. A factor analytic study of menopausal symptoms in middle aged women. *Indian Journal of Clinical Psychology* 7:125–128.

James, G. D., Broege, P. A., and Schlussel, Y. R. 1996. Assessing cardiovascular risk and stress-related blood pressure variability in young women employed in wage jobs. *American Journal of Human Biology* 8:743–749.

James, G. D., and Brown, D. E. 1997. The biological stress response and lifestyle: catecholamines and blood pressure. *Annual Review of Anthropology* 26:313–315.

James, G. D., and Marion, R. M. 1994. Cardiovascular differences by phase of the menstrual cycle. *Collegium Anthropologicum* 18:63–71.

Jamison, C. S., Cornell, L. L., Jamison, P. L., and Nakazato, H. 2002. Are all grandmothers equal? A review and a preliminary test of the "grandmother hypothesis" in Tokugawa Japan. *American Journal of Physical Anthropology* 119:67–76.

Jaszmann, L. 1973. Epidemiology of climacteric and post-climacteric complaints. *Frontiers of Hormone Research* 2:22–34.

Jaszmann, L., van Lith, N. D., and Zaat, J.C.A. 1969. The age at menopause in the Netherlands: the statistical analysis of a survey. *International Journal of Fertility* 14:106–117.

Jick, H., Parker, J., and Morrison, A. S. 1977. Relation between smoking and age of natural menopause. *Lancet* 1:1354–1355.

Johnson, J., Canning, J., Kaneko, T., Pru, J. K., and Tilly, J. L. 2004. Germline stem cells and follicular renewal in the postnatal mammalian ovary. *Nature* 428:145–150.

Johnson, R. L., and Kapsalis, E. 1998. Menopause in free-ranging rhesus macaques: estimated incidence, relation to body condition, and adaptive significance. *International Journal of Primatology* 19(4):751–765.

Johnston, S. L. 2001. Associations with age at natural menopause in Blackfeet women. *American Journal of Human Biology* 13:512–520.

Jordan, B. 1993. *Birth in Four Cultures.* Prospect Heights, IL: Waveland Press.

Junod, H. A. 1927. *The Life of a South African Tribe.* vol. I. London: Macmillan and Co.

Kaiser, F. E., Morley, J. E., and Korenman, S. G. 1993. Hypothalamic function and its relationship to impotence. In F. Haseltine, C. A. Paulsen, and C. Wang, eds., *Reproductive Issues and the Aging Male, 77–87.* AAAS Publication 93-22S, Washington, DC.

Kaplan, H., Hill, K., Lancaster, J., and Hurtado, A. M. 2000. A theory of human life history evolution: diet, intelligence, and longevity. *Evolutionary Anthropology* 9:156–185.

Kaufert, P. 1988. Menopause as process or event: the creation of definitions in biomedicine. In M. Lock and D. R. Gordon, eds., *Biomedicine Examined, 331–349.* Boston: Kluwar Academic Publishers.

Kaufert, P., and Gilbert, P. 1986. Women, menopause, and medicalization. *Culture, Medicine and Psychology* 10(1):7–21.

Kaufert, P., Gilbert, P., and Tate, R. 1987. Defining menopausal status: the impact of longitudinal data. *Maturitas* 9:217–226.

———. 1992. The Manitoba Project: a re-examination of the link between menopause and depression. *Maturitas* 14:143–155.

Kaufert, P. A., and Lock, M. 1997. Medicalization of women's third age. *Journal of Psychosomatic Obstetrics and Gynecology* 18:81–86.

Kaufert, P., Lock, M., McKinlay, S., Beyene, Y., Coope, J., Davis, D., Eliasson, M., Gognalons-Nicolet, M., Goodman, M., and Holte, A. 1986. Menopause research: the Korpilampi workshop. *Social Science and Medicine* 22(11):1285–1289.

Kaufert, P., and Syrotuik, J. 1981. Symptom reporting at the menopause. *Social Science and Medicine* 15E:173–184.

Kaufman, F. R., Kought, M. D., Donnell, G. N., Goebelsmann, U., March, C., and Koch, R. 1981. Hypergonadotropic hypogonadism in female patients with galactosemia. *New England Journal of Medicine* 304:994–998.

Kaufman, H. K. 1960. *Banbkhuad: A Community Study in Thailand.* Monograph 10. Locust Valley, NY: Association for Asian Studies.

Kelsey, J. L., Gammon, M. D., and John, E. M. 1993. Reproductive factors and breast cancer. *Epidemiologic Reviews* 15:36–47.

Kennedy, D. L., Baum, C., and Forbes, M. B. 1985. Noncontraceptive estrogens and progestins: use patterns over time. *Obstetrics and Gynecology* 65:441–446.

Kerns, R. D., Haythornthwaite, J., Southwick, S., and Giller, E. L. 1990. The role of marital interaction in chronic pain and depressive symptom severity. *Journal of Psychosomatic Research* 34(4):401–408.

Kirchengast, S. 1993. Relations between anthropometric characteristics and degree of severity of the climacteric syndrome in Austrian women. *Maturitas* 17:167–180.

Kirchengast, S., Hartmann, B., and Huber, J. 1996. Serum levels of sex hormones, thyroid hormones, growth hormone, IGF I, and cortisol and their relations to body fat distribution in healthy women dependent on their menopausal status. *Zeitschrift für Morphologie und Anthropologie* 81(2):223–234.

Kirkwood, T.B.L. 1985. Comparative and evolutionary aspects of longevity. In C. E. Finch, and E. L. Schneider, eds., *Handbook of the Biology of Aging,* 27–44. New York: Van Nostrand Reinhold.

Kirz, D. S., Dorchester, W., and Freeman, R. K. 1985. Advanced maternal age: the mature gravida. *American Journal of Obstetrics and Gynecology* 152(1):7–12.

Kjerulff, K., Langenberg, P., and Guzinski, G. 1993. The socioeconomic correlates of hysterectomies in the United States. *American Journal of Public Health* 83(1):106–108.

Kjerulff, K., Langenberg, P., Seidman, J. D., Stolley, P. D., and Guzinski, G. M. 1996. Racial differences in severity, symptoms, and age at diagnosis. *Journal of Reproductive Medicine* 41:483–490.

Kleinman, A. 1995. *Writing at the Margin: Discourse between Anthropology and Medicine.* Berkeley: University of California Press.

Kletzky, O. A., and Borenstein, R. 1987. Vasomotor instability of the menopause. In D. R. Mishell, ed., *Menopause: Physiology and Pharmacology,* 53–65. Chicago: Year Book Medical.

Kline, J., and Levin, B. 1992. Trisomy and age at menopause: predicted associations given a link with rate of oocyte atresia. *Paediatric and Perinatal Epidemiology* 6:225–239.

Knight, D. C., Lyons Wall, P., and Eden, J. A. 1996. A review of phytoestrogens and their effects in relation to menopausal symptoms. *Australian Journal of Nutrition and Dietetics* 53:5–11.

Kohn, R. R. 1978. *Principles of Mammalian Aging.* Englewood Cliffs, NJ: Prentice-Hall.

Kolata, G. 1997. A record and big questions as woman gives birth at 63. *New York Times,* April 24:AI, A25.

Komesaroff, P. P., Rothfield, P., and Daly, J. 1997. *Reinterpreting Menopause: Cultural and Philosophical Issues.* London: Routledge.

Korenman, S. G., Sherman, B. M., and Korenman, J. C. 1978. Reproductive hormone function: the perimenopausal period and beyond. *Clinical Endocrinology and Metabolism.* 7(3):625–643.

Kormondy, E. J., and Brown, D. E. 1998. *Fundamentals of Human Ecology.* Upper Saddle River, NJ: Prentice Hall.

Krauss, C. M., Turksoy, R. N., Atkins, L., McLaughlin, C., Brown, L. G., and Page, D. C. 1987. Familial premature ovarian failure due to an interstitial deletion of the long arm of the X chromosome. *New England Journal of Medicine* 317(3):125–131.

Kronenberg, F. L. 1990. Hot flashes: epidemiology and physiology. *Annals of the New York Academy of Sciences* 592:52–86.

———. 1994. Hot flashes: phenomenology, quality of life, and search for treatment options. *Experimental Gerontology* 29(3–4):319–336.

Kronenberg, F., and Barnard, R. M. 1992. Modulation of menopausal hot flashes by ambient temperature. *Journal of Thermal Biology* 17:43–49.

Kuh, D., and Hardy, R. 2002. *A Life Course Approach to Women's Health.* New York: Oxford University Press.

Kuh, D., Hardy, R., Rodgers, B., and Wadsworth, M.E.J. 2002. Lifetime risk factors for women's psychological distress in midlife. *Social Science and Medicine* 55(11):1957–1973.

Kuh, D. L., Wadsworth, M., and Hardy, R. 1997. Women's health in midlife: the influence of the menopause, social factors, and health in earlier life. *British Journal of Obstetrics and Gynaecology* 104(8):923–933.

Kupperman, H. S., Blatt, M.H.G., Wiesbader, H., and Filler, W. 1953. Comparative clinical evaluation of estrogenic preparations by the menopausal and amenorrheal indices. *Journal of Clinical Endocrinology and Metabolism* 13:688–703.

Kvale, G., and Heuch, I. 1988. Menstrual factors and breast cancer risk. *Cancer* 62:1625–1631.

Kwawukume, E. Y., Ghosh, T. S., and Wilson, J. B. 1993. Menopausal age of Ghanian women. *International Journal of Gynaecology and Obstetrics* 40:151–155.

LaBarbera, A. R., Miller, M. M., Ober, C., and Rebar, R. W. 1988. Autoimmune etiology in premature ovarian failure. *American Journal of Reproductive Immunology and Microbiology* 16:115–122.

Lahdenperä, M., Lummaa, V., Helle, S., Tremblay, M., and Russell, A. F. 2004. Fitness benefits of prolonged post-reproductive lifespan in women. *Nature* 428:178–181.

Lancaster, J. B., and King, B. J. 1992. An evolutionary perspective on menopause. In V. Kerns, and J. K. Brown, eds., *In Her Prime: New Views of Middle-Aged Women,* 7–15. South Hadley, MA: Bergin and Garvey.

Lancaster, J. B., and Lancaster, C. S. 1983. The parental investment: the hominid adaptation. In D. J. Ortner, ed., *How Humans Adapt: A Biocultural Odyssey,* 33–65. Washington, DC: Smithsonian Institution Press.

Lansac, J. 1995. Delayed parenting. Is delayed childbearing a good thing? *Human Reproduction* 10(5):1033–1035.

Lapin, B. A., Krilova, R. I., Cherkovich, G., and Asanov, S. 1979. Observations from Sukhumi. In D. Bowden, ed., *Aging in Nonhuman Primates,* 183–202. New York: Van Nostrand Reinhold.

Laumann, E. O., Paik, A., and Rosen, R. C. 1999. Sexual dysfunction in the United States: prevalence and predictors. *Journal of the American Medical Association* 281:537–544.

Leatherman, T. L., and Goodman, A. H. 1997. Expanding the biocultural synthesis toward a biology of poverty. *American Journal of Physical Anthropology* 102(1):1–3.

Lee, E. T. 1980. *Statistical Methods for Survival Data Analysis*. Belmont, CA: Lifetime Learning Publications.

Lee, S. G. 1958. Social influences in Zulu dreaming. *Journal of Social Psychology* 47:265–283.

Lee, S. J., Lenton, E. A., Sexton, L., and Cooke, I. D. 1988. The effect of age on the cyclical patterns of plasma LH, FSH, oestradiol and progesterone in women with regular menstrual cycles. *Human Reproduction* 3(7):851–855.

Leidy, L. 1991. The timing of menopause in biological and socio-cultural context: a lifespan approach. Ph.D. diss., State University of New York at Albany.

———. 1994a. Biological aspects of menopause: across the lifespan. *Annual Review of Anthropology* 23:231–253.

———. 1994b. The possible role of the pessary in the etiology of toxic shock. *Medical Anthropology Quarterly* 8(2):198–208.

———. 1996a. The lifespan approach to the study of human biology: an introduction. *American Journal of Human Biology* 8(6):699–702.

———. 1996b. The timing of menopause in relation to body size and weight change. *Human Biology* 68(6):997–1012.

———. 1996c. Symptoms of menopause in relation to the timing of reproductive events and past menstrual experience. *American Journal of Human Biology* 8:761–769.

———. 1997. Menopausal symptoms and everyday complaints. *Menopause* 4(3):154–160.

———. 1998. Menarche, menopause, and migration: implications for breast cancer research. *American Journal of Human Biology* 10(4):451–457.

———. 1999a. Menopause in evolutionary perspective. In W. R. Trevathan, E. O. Smith, and J. J. McKenna, eds., *Evolutionary Medicine*, 407–427. New York: Oxford University Press.

———. 1999b. The effect of exclusion: rates of hysterectomy and comparisons of age at natural menopause. *American Journal of Human Biology* 11:687–693.

Leidy, L., Canali, C., and Callahan, W. 2000. The medicalization of menopause: implications for recruitment of study participants. *Menopause* 7(3):193–199.

Leidy, L., Godfrey, L., and Sutherland, M. 1998. Is follicular atresia biphasic? *Fertility and Sterility* 70(5):851–859.

Leidy Sievert, L. 2001. Menopause in Puebla, Mexico: fieldwork details and preliminary results. *Association for Anthropology and Gerontology Newsletter* 22(3):9–10.

Leidy Sievert, L. 2003. El envejecimiento reproductivo: la menopausia en Puebla, Mexico. *Estudios de Antropología Biológica*. 11:91–112.

Leidy Sievert, L., Waddle, D., and Canali, K. 2001. Marital status and age at natural menopause: considering pheromonal influence. *American Journal of Human Biology* 13:479–485.

Lepine, L. A., Hillis, S. D., Marchbanks, P. A., Koonin, L. M., Morrow, B., Kieke, B. A., and Wilcox, L. S. 1997. Hysterectomy surveillance—United States, 1980–1993. *Morbidity and Mortality Weekly Report*, CDC Surveillance Summaries, 46(4):1–15.

Levran, D., Ben-Shlomo, I., Dor, J., Ben-Rafael, Z., Nebel, L., and Mashiach, S. 1991. Aging of endometrium and oocytes: observations on conception and abortion rates in an egg donation model. *Fertility and Sterility* 56:1091–1094.

Linde, R., Doelle, G. C., Alexander, N., Kirchner, F., Vale, W., Rivier, J., and Rabin, D. 1981. Reversible inhibition of testicular steroidogenesis and spermatogenesis by a potent gonadotropin releasing hormone agonist in normal men: an approach toward the development of a male contraceptive. *New England Journal of Medicine* 305:663–667.

Lindquist, O., Bengtsson, C., Hansson, T., and Jonsson, R. 1983. Changes in bone mineral content of the axial skeleton in relation to aging and the menopause. *Scandinavian Journal of Clinical and Laboratory Investigation* 43:333–338.

Lock, M. 1986. Ambiguities of aging: Japanese experience and perceptions of menopause. *Culture, Medicine, and Psychiatry* 10(1):23–46.

———. 1991. Contested meanings of the menopause. *Lancet* 337(8752):1270–1272.

———. 1993. *Encounters with Aging: Mythologies of Menopause in Japan and North America.* Berkeley: University of California Press.

———. 1998. Menopause: lessons from anthropology. *Psychosomatic Medicine* 60:410–419.

———. 2005. Cross-cultural vasomotor symptom reporting: conceptual and methodological issues [editorial]. *Menopause* 12(3):239–241.

Lock, M., and Kaufert, P. 2001. Menopause, local biologies, and cultures of aging. *American Journal of Human Biology* 13:494–504.

Lock, M., and Scheper-Hughes, N. 1996. A critical-interpretive approach in medical anthropology: rituals and routines of discipline and dissent. In C. F. Sargent and T. M. Johnson, eds., *Medical Anthropology: Contemporary Theory and Method,* 41–70. Westport, CT: Praeger.

Longcope, C., Franz, C., Morello, C., Baker, R., and Johnston, C. C. 1986. Steroid and gonadotropin levels in women during the perimenopausal years. *Maturitas* 8:189–196.

Lovejoy, C. O. 1981. The origin of man. *Science* 211:341–350.

Lu, L.-J.W., Tice, J. A., and Bellino, F. L. 2001. Phytoestrogens and healthy aging: gaps in knowledge. A workshop report. *Menopause* 8(3):157–170.

Luborsky, J., Llanes, B., Davies, S., Binor, Z., Radwanska, E., and Pong, R. 1999. Ovarian autoimmunity: greater frequency of autoantibodies in premature menopause and unexplained infertility than in the general population. *Clinical Immunology* 90(3):368–374.

Luoto, R., Kaprio, J., and Uutela, A. 1994. Age at natural menopause and sociodemographic status in Finland. *American Journal of Epidemiology* 139:64–76.

MacMahon, B., and Worcester, J. 1966. *Age at Menopause: United States, 1960–1962.* National Center for Health Statistics Series 11(19), Department of Health, Education, and Welfare.

MacPherson, K. I. 1985. Osteoporosis and menopause: a feminist analysis of the social construction of a syndrome. *Advances in Nursing Science* 7(4):11–22.

Malacara, H.J.M. 1998. Epidemiología. In S. Carranza Lira, ed., *Atención integral del climaterio,* 5–17. Mexico, D. F., Mexico: McGraw-Hill Interamericana.

Mall, A., Shirk, G., and Van Voorhis, B. J. 2002. Previous tubal ligation is a risk factor for hysterectomy after rollerball endometrial ablation. *Obstetrics and Gynecology* 100(4):659–664.

Mansfield, P. K., and Bracken, S. J. 2003. *Tremin: A History of the World's Oldest Ongoing Study of Menstruation and Women's Health.* Lemont, PA: East Rim Publishers.

Mansfield, P. K., Carey, M., Anderson, A., Barsom, S., and Koch, P. B. 2003. Tracking women's changing menstrual status across the menopausal transition: Tremin research program data. Fifteenth Biennial Conference of the Society for Menstrual Cycle Research, June 5–7.

Manson, J. E., Hsia, J., Johnson, K. C., et al., for the Women's Health Initiative Investigators. 2003. Estrogen plus progestin and the risk of coronary heart disease. *New England Journal of Medicine* 349:523–534.

Marks, J. 1995. *Human Biodiversity: Genes, Race, and History.* New York: Aldine de Gruyter.

Marks, N. F., and Shinberg, D. S. 1997. Socioeconomic differences in hysterectomy: the Wisconsin Longitudinal Study. *American Journal of Public Health* 87(9):507–514.

Maroulis, G. B. 1991. Effect of aging on fertility and pregnancy. *Seminars in Reproductive Endocrinology* 9(3):165–175.

Marsh, H., and Kasuya, T. 1986. Evidence for reproductive senescence in female cetaceans. *Report of the International Whaling Commission* 8:57–74.

Marshall, L. M., Spiegelman, D., Barbieri, R., Goldman, M., Manson, J., Colditz, G. A., Willett, W. C., and Hunter, D. J. 1997. Variation in the incidence of uterine leiomyoma among premenopausal women by age and race. *Obstetrics and Gynecology* 90:967–973.

Martin, C. R. 1985. *Endocrine Physiology.* New York: Oxford University Press.

Martin, E. 1987. *The Woman in the Body.* Boston: Beacon Press.

Martin, M. C., Block, J. E., Sanchez, S. D., Arnaud, C. D., and Beyene, Y. 1993. Menopause without symptoms: the endocrinology of menopause among rural Mayan Indians. *American Journal of Obstetrics and Gynecology* 168:1839–1845.

Matthews, K. A., Sowers, M. F., Derby, C. A., Stein, E., Miracle-McMahill, H., Crawford, S. L., and Pasternak, R. C. 2005. Ethnic differences in cardiovascular risk factor burden among middle-aged women: Study of Women's Health Across the Nation (SWAN). *American Heart Journal* 149(6):1066–1073.

Matthews, K. A., Wing, R. R., Kuller, L. H., Meilahn, E. N., Kelsey, S. F., Costello, E. J., and Caggiula, A. W. 1990. Influences of natural menopause on psychological characteristics and symptoms of middle-aged healthy women. *Journal of Consulting and Clinical Psychology* 58:345–351.

Mattison, D. R., Evans, M. I., Schwimmer, W. B., White, B. J., Jensen, B., and Schulman, J. D. 1984. Familial premature ovarian failure. *American Journal of Human Genetics* 36(6):1341–1348.

Mattison, D. R., Plowchalk, D. R., Meadows, M. J., Miller, M. M., Malek, A., and London, S. 1989. The effect of smoking on oogenesis, fertilization, and implantation. *Seminars in Reproductive Endocrinology* 7:291–304.

Mattison, D. R., and Thomford, P. J. 1987. The effect of smoking on reproductive ability and reproductive lifespan. In M. J. Rosenberg, ed., *Smoking and Reproductive Health*, 47–54. Littleton, MA: PSG Publishing Company.

Mattison, D. R., and Thorgeirsson, S. 1978. Smoking and industrial pollution and their effects on menopause and ovarian cancer. *Lancet* 1:187–188.

Mayer, P. J. 1982. Evolutionary advantage of the menopause. *Human Ecology* 10:477–494.

McCrea, F. B. 1983. The politics of menopause: the "discovery" of a deficiency disease. *Social Problems* 31(1):111–123.

McDonough, P. G. 1999. Factoring in complexity and oocyte memory—can transformations and cyperpathology distort reality?' [editorial comment]. *Fertility and Sterility* 71:1172–1174.

McElroy, A. 1990. Bicultural models in studies of human health and adaptation. *Medical Anthropology Quarterly* 4(3):243–265.

McElroy, A., and Townsend, P. K. 2004. *Medical Anthropology in Ecological Perspective,* 4th ed. Boulder Westview Press.

McKinlay, S. M., Brambilla, D. J., and Posner, J. G. 1992. The normal menopause transition. *American Journal of Human Biology* 4:37–46.

McKinlay, S. M., and Jefferys, M. 1974. The menopausal syndrome. *British Journal of Preventative and Social Medicine* 28:108–115.

McKinlay, S. M., Jefferys, M., and Thompson, B. 1972. An investigation of the age at menopause. *Journal of Biosocial Science* 4:161–173.

McKinlay, S. M., and McKinlay, J. B. 1973. Selected studies of the menopause—a methodological critique. *Journal of Biosocial Science* 5:533–555.

McKinlay, J. B., McKinlay, S. M., and Brambilla, D. 1987. The relative contributions of endocrine changes and social circumstances to depression in mid-aged women. *Journal of Health and Social Behavior* 28:345–363.

McMahon, B., Trichopoulos, D., Cole, P., and Brown, J. 1982. Cigarette smoking and urinary estrogens. *New England Journal of Medicine* 307:1062–1065.

McPherson, K., Wennberg, J. E., Hovid, O. B., and Clifford, P. 1982. Small-area variations in the use of common surgical procedures: an international comparison of New England, England, and Norway. *New England Journal of Medicine* 307:1310–1314.

Meilahn, E. N., Matthews, K. A., Egeland, G., and Kelsey, S. F. 1989. Characteristics of women with hysterectomy. *Maturitas* 11(4):319–329.

Meites, J., Huang, H., Simpkins, J., and Steger, R. 1982. Central nervous system neurotransmitters during the decline of reproductive activity. In P. Fiorette, L. Martini, G. Melis, and S. Yen, eds., *The Menopause: Clinical, Endocrinological, and Pathophysiological Aspects*, 3–13. New York: Academic Press.

Meites, J., and Lu, J.K.H. 1994. Reproductive ageing and neuroendocrine function. *Oxford Reviews of Reproductive Biology* 16:215–247.

Melby, M. K. 2005. Vasomotor symptom prevalence and language of menopause in Japan. *Menopause* 12(3):250–257.

Melby, M. K., Lock, M., and Kaufert, P. 2005. Culture and symptom reporting at menopause. *Human Reproduction Update* 11(5):495–512.

Meldrum, D. R. 1993. Female reproductive ageing—ovarian and uterine factors. *Fertility and Sterility* 59:1–5.

Mendelson, J. H., Cristofaro, P., Ellingboe, J., Benedikt, R., and Mello, N. K. 1985. Acute effects of marihuana on luteinizing hormone in menopausal women. *Pharmacology, Biochemistry and Behavior* 23:765–768.

Mercer, R. T., Nichols, E. G., and Doyle, G. C. 1989. *Transitions in a Woman's Life: Major Life Events in Developmental Context*. New York: Springer.

Merchant, K. M., and Kurz, K. M. 1993. Women's nutrition through the life cycle: social and biological vulnerabilities. In M. Koblinsky, J. Timyan, and J. Gay, eds., *The Health of Women: A Global Perspective*, 63–90. Boulder: Westview Press.

Merry, B. J., and Holehan, A. M. 1994. Aging of the female reproductive system: the menopause. In P. S. Timiras, ed., *Physiological Basis of Aging and Geriatrics*, 2nd ed., 147–170. Ann Arbor, Mich.: CRC Press.

Messenger, J. C. 1971. Sex and repression in an Irish folk community. In D. S. Marshall and R. C. Suggs, eds., *Human Sexual Behavior: Variations in the Ethnographic Spectrum*, 3–37. Studies in Sex and Society Series. New York: Basic Books.

Metcalf, M. G., Donald, R. A., and Livesey, J. H. 1981. Pituitary-ovarian function in normal women during the menopausal transition. *Clinical Endocrinology* 14:245–255.

Mishell, D. R. 1989. Estrogen replacement therapy: an overview. *Obstetrics and Gynecology* 161:1825–1827.

Mitchell, E. S., Woods, N. F., and Mariella, A. 2000. Three stages of the menopausal transition from the Seattle Midlife Women's Health Study: toward a more precise definition. *Menopause* 7(5):334–339.

———. 2003. FSH and estrone patterns during the menopausal transition [abstract], fifteenth Biennial Conference of the Society for Menstrual Cycle Research, June 5–7.

Molnar, G. W. 1975. Body temperature during menopausal hot flashes. *Journal of Applied Physiology* 38:499–503.

———. 1981. Menopausal hot flashes: their cycles and relation to air temperature. *Obstetrics and Gynecology* (supp.) 57:52–55.

Molnar, S. 2002. *Human Variation: Races, Types, and Ethnic Groups.* 5th ed. Englewood Cliffs, NJ: Prentice Hall.

Moore, B., and Kombe, H. 1991. Climacteric symptoms in a Tanzanian community. *Maturitas* 13:229–234.

Moore, K. L. 1988. *Essentials of Human Embryology.* Philadelphia: B. C. Decker.

Moore, L. G., Van Arsdale, P., Glittenberg, J., and Aldrich, R. 1980. *The Biocultural Basis of Health.* Prospect Heights, IL: Waveland Press.

Morabia, A., Costanza, M. C., and WHO Collaborative. 1998. International variability in ages at menarche, first livebirth, and menopause. *American Journal of Epidemiology* 148(12):1195–1205.

Mori, T. 1994. Post-menopausal pregnancy is permissible for women below 60 years of age. *Human Reproduction* 9(2):187.

Morris, J. 1938. *Living with Lepchas: A book about the Sikkam, Himalayas.* London: W. Heinemann.

Mort, E. A., Weissman, J. S., and Epstein, A. M. 1994. Physician discretion and racial variation in the use of surgical procedures. *Archives of Internal Medicine* 154(7):761–767.

Mueller, K. A., Jiménez Zerón Sánchez, G., and Leidy Sievert, L. 2003. Sources of information and HRT prescribing practices among gynecologists in Puebla, Mexico. *Maturitas* 45:137–144.

Murdock, G. P., Ford, C. S., Hudson, A. E., Kennedy, R., Simmons, L. W., and Whiting, J.W.M. 1982. *Outline of Cultural Materials,* 5th ed. New Haven, CT: Human Relations Area Files.

Murphy, L. L., Muñoz, R. M., Adrian, B. A., and Villanúa, M. A. 1998. Function of cannabinoid receptors in the neuroendocrine regulation of hormone secretion. *Neurobiology of Disease* 5:432–446.

Nachtigall, L., and Heilman, J. R. 1986. *Estrogen: The Facts Can Change Your Life.* Los Angeles: Price Stern Sloan.

Naeye, R. L. 1983. Maternal age, obstetric complications, and the outcome of pregnancy. *Obstetrics and Gynecology* 61(2):210–216.

Naftolin, F., Whitten, P., and Keefe, D. 1994. An evolutionary perspective on the climacteric and menopause. *Menopause* 1(4):223–225.

Nagata, C., Shimizu, H., Takami, R., Hayashi, M., Takeda, N., and Yasuda, K. 1999. Hot flushes and other menopausal symptoms in relation to soy product intake in Japanese women. *Climacteric* 2:6–12.

Nass, T. E., Lapolt, P. S., and Lu, J.K.H. 1982. Effects of prolonged caging with fertile males on reproductive functions in aging female rats. *Biology of Reproduction* 27:609–615.

Navot, D., Bergh, P. A., Williams, M. A., Garrisa, G. J., Guzman, I., Sandler, B., and Grunfeld, L. 1991. Poor oocyte quality rather than implantation failure as a cause of age-related decline in female fertility. *Lancet* 337:1375–1377.

Nelson, J. F., and Felicio, L. S. 1985. Reproductive aging in the female: an etiological perspective. In M. Rothstein, ed., *Review of Biological Research in Aging,* vol. 2, 251–314. New York: Alan R. Liss.

Neri, A., Bider, D., Lidor, U., and Ovadia, J. 1982. Menopausal age in various ethnic groups in Israel. *Maturitas* 4:341–348.

Neslihan Carda, S., Atike Bilge, S., Nilgun Ozturk, T., Oya, G., Ece, O., and Hamiyet, B. 1998. The menopausal age, related factors, and climacteric symptoms in Turkish women. *Maturitas* 30:37–40.

Nesse, R. M., and Williams, G. C. 1994. *Why We Get Sick: The New Science of Darwinian Medicine.* New York: Vintage Books.

Neugarten, B. 1969. Continuities and discontinuities of psychological issues into adult lives. *Human Development* 12:121–130.

———. 1996. The aging society and my academic life. In D. A. Neugarten, ed., *The Meanings of Age: Selected Papers of Bernice L. Neugarten,* 1–16. Chicago: University of Chicago Press.

Neugarten, B., and Datan, N. 1973. Sociological perspectives on the life cycle. In P. B. Baltes, and K. W. Schaie, eds., *Life-Span Developmental Psychology: Personality and Socialization,* 53–79. New York: Academic Press.

———. 1974. The middle years. In S. Arieti, ed., *American Handbook of Psychiatry,* 2nd ed., vol. 1: *The Foundations of Psychiatry,* 592–608. New York: Basic Books.

Neugarten, B., and Kraines, R. 1965. Menopausal symptoms in women of various ages. *Psychosomatic Medicine* 27:266–273.

Neugarten, B., Wood, V., Kraines, R. J., and Loomis, B. 1963. Women's attitudes toward the menopause. *Vita Humana* 6:140–151.

Nevitt, M., Cummings, S., Lane, N., Hochzung, M. C., Scott, J. C., Pressman, A. R., Gerant, H., and Cauley, J. A. 1996. Association of estrogen replacement therapy with the risk of osteoarthritis of the hip in elderly white women. *Archives of Internal Medicine* 156:2073–2080.

New York State Department of Health. 1988. *Hysterectomies in New York State: A Statistical Profile.* Information Systems and Health Statistics Group, New York State Department of Health, June.

Nichols, S. M., Bavister, B. D., Brenner, C. A., Didier, P. J., Harrison, R. M., and Kubisch, H. M. 2005. Ovarian senescence in the rhesus monkey *(Macaca mulatta). Human Reproduction* 20(1):79–83.

Nishida, T., Corp, N., Hamai, M., Hasegawa, T., Hiraiwa-Hasegawa, M., Hosaka, K., Hunt, K. D., Itoh, N., Kawanaka, K., Matsumoto-Oda, A., Mitani, J. C., Nakamura, M., Norikoshi, K., Sakamaki, T., Turner, L., Uehara, S., and Zamma, K. 2003. Demography, female life history, and reproductive profiles among the chimpanzees of Mahale. *American Journal of Primatology* 59:99–121.

Nishida, T., Takasaki, H., and Takahata, Y. 1990. Demography and reproductive profiles. In T. Nishida, ed., *The Chimpanzees of the Mahale Mountains: Sexual and Life History Strategies,* 63–97. Tokyo: University of Tokyo Press.

Notelovitz, M. 1989. Hormonal therapy in climacteric women: compliance and its socio-economic impact. *Public Health Reports Supplement* (Sept.–Oct.): 70–75.

Notman, M. T. 1980. Changing roles for women at mid-life. In W. Norman, and T. Scramella, eds., *Mid-Life: Developmental and Clinical Issues*, 85–109. New York: Brunner/Mazel.

Novak, E. R. 1970. Ovulation after fifty. *Obstetrics and Gynecology* 36:903–910.

Nuti, R., and Martini, G. 1993. Effects of age and menopause on bone density of entire skeleton in healthy and osteoporotic women. *Osteoporosis International* 3:59–65.

Obermeyer, C. M. 2000. Menopause across cultures: a review of the evidence. *Menopause* 7:184–192.

Obermeyer, C. M., Ghorayeb, F., and Reynolds, R. 1999. Symptom reporting around the menopause in Beirut, Lebanon. *Maturitas* 33:249–258.

O'Connell, J. F., Hawkes, K., and Blurton Jones, N. G. 1999. Grandmothering and the evolution of *Homo erectus*. *Journal of Human Evolution* 36:461–485.

O'Connor, K. A., Holman, D. J., and Wood, J. W. 1998. Declining fecundity and ovarian ageing in natural fertility populations. *Maturitas* 30:127–136.

O'Connor, V. M., Del Mar, C. B., Sheehan, M., Siskind, V., Fox-Young, S., and Cragg, C. 1995. Do psycho-social factors contribute more to symptom reporting by middle-aged women than hormonal status? *Maturitas* 20:63–69.

Okonofua, F. E., Lawal, A., and Bamgbose, J. K. 1990. Features of menopause and menopausal age in Nigerian women. *International Journal of Gynecology and Obstetrics* 31: 341–345.

Oktay, K. 2001. Ovarian tissue cryopreservation and transplantation: preliminary findings and implications for cancer patients. *Human Reproduction Update* 7:526–534.

Oktay, K., and Karlikaya, G. 2000. Ovarian function after transplantation of frozen, banked autologous ovarian tissue. *New England Journal of Medicine* 342(25):1919.

Oktay, K., and Sonmezer, M. 2004. Fertility preservation not just ovarian cryopreservation. *Human Reproduction* 19:1–4.

Olazábal Ulacia, J. C., García Paniagua, R., Montero Luengo, J., García Gutiérrez, J. F., Sendín Melguizo, P. P., and Holgado Sánchez, M. A. 1999. Models of intervention in menopause: proposal of a holistic or integral model. *Menopause* 6(3):264–272.

Oldenhave, A., and Jaszmann, L.J.B. 1991. The climacteric: absence or presence of hot flushes and their relation to other complaints. In E. Schonbaum, ed., *The Climacteric Hot Flush*. Progress in Basic and Clinical Pharmacology, 6:6–39. Basel: Karger.

Oldenhave, A., Jaszmann, L.J.B., Haspels, A. A., and Everaerd, W.T.A.M. 1993. Impact of climacteric on well-being: a survey based on 5213 women 39 to 60 years old. *American Journal of Obstetrics and Gynecology* 168:772–780.

O'Rourke, M. T., and Ellison, P. T. 1993. Menopause and ovarian senescence in human females. *American Journal of Physical Anthropology* (supp.) 16:154.

Ortiz, A. P., Harlow, S., Sowers, M., and Romaguera, J. 2003. Age at natural menopause in a sample of Puerto Rican women. *Puerto Rican Health Sciences Journal* 22(4):337–342.

Ossewaarde, M. E., Bots, M. L., Verbeek, A. L., Peeters, P. H., van der Graaf, Y., Grobbee, D. E., and van der Schouw, Y. T. 2005. Age at menopause, cause-specific mortality, and total life expectancy. *Epidemiology* 16(4):556–562.

Ottenberg, P. V. 1958. Marriage relationships in the double descent system of the Afikpo Igbo of Southeast Nigeria. Ph.D. diss., Northwestern University.

Palmlund, I. 1997a. The marketing of estrogens for menopausal and postmenopausal women. *Journal of Psychosomatic Obstetrics and Gynecology* 18:158–164.

———. 1997b. The social construction of menopause as risk. *Journal of Psychosomatic Obstetrics and Gynecology* 18:87–94.

Panter-Brick, C. 2002. Sexual division of labor: energetic and evolutionary scenarios. *American Journal of Human Biology* 14:627–640.

Panter-Brick, C., and Pollard, T. M. 1999. Work and hormonal variation in subsistence and industrial contexts. In C. Panter-Brick, and C. M. Worthman, eds., *Hormones, Health, and Behavior: A Socio-Ecological and Lifespan Perspective,* 139–183. Cambridge: Cambridge University Press.

Parazzini, F., Negri, E., and La Vecchia, C. 1992. Reproductive and general lifestyle determinants of age at menopause. *Maturitas* 15:141–149.

Parra-Cabrera, S., Hernandez-Avila, M., Tamayo-y-Orozco, J., López-Carrillo, L., and Meneses-González, F. 1996. Exercise and reproductive factors as predictors of bone density among osteoporotic women in Mexico City. *Calcified Tissue International* 59:89–94.

Partridge, L., and Harvey, P. H. 1988. The ecological context of life history evolution. *Science* 241:1449–1455.

Paulson, R. J., Thornton, M. H., Francis, M. M., and Salvador, H. S. 1997. Successful pregnancy in a 63-year-old woman. *Fertility and Sterility* 67(5):949–951.

Pavelka, M. S., and Fedigan, L. M. 1991. Menopause: a comparative life history perspective. *Yearbook of Physical Anthropology* 34:13–38.

——. 1999. Reproductive termination in female Japanese monkeys: a comparative life history perspective. *American Journal of Physical Anthropology* 109:455–464.

Pavlik, E. J., DePriest, P. D., Gallion, H. H., Ueland, F. R., Reedy, M. B., Kryscio, R. J., and van Nagell, J. R., Jr. 2000. Ovarian volume related to age. *Gynecologic Oncology* 77(3):410–412.

Payer, L. 1987. *How to Avoid a Hysterectomy.* New York: Pantheon Books.

——. 1988. *Medicine and Culture: Varieties of Treatment in the United States, England, West Germany, and France.* New York: Henry Holt and Company.

Peacock, N. 1991. An evolutionary perspective on the patterning of maternal investment in pregnancy. *Human Nature* 2:351–385.

Pearlstein, T. B. 1995. Hormones and depression: what are the facts about premenstrual syndrome, menopause, and hormone replacement therapy? *American Journal of Obstetrics and Gynecology* 173:646–653.

Peccei, J. S. 1995. A hypothesis for the origin and evolution of menopause. *Maturitas* 21:83–89.

——. 1999. First estimates of heritability in the age of menopause. *Current Anthropology* 40:553–558.

——. 2001. A critique of the grandmother hypothesis: old and new. *American Journal of Human Biology* 13:434–452.

Peters, H., and McNatty, K. P. 1980. *The Ovary: A Correlation of Structure and Function in Mammals.* New York: Granada.

Peterson, H. B., Jeng, G., Folger, S. G., Hillis, S. A., Marchbanks, P. A., and Wilcox, L. S. for The U.S. Collaborative Review of Sterilization Working Group 2000. The risk of menstrual abnormalities after tubal sterilization. *New England Journal of Medicine* 343(23):1681–1687.

Pike, I. L. 1999. Age, reproductive history, seasonality, and maternal body composition during pregnancy for nomadic Turkana pastoralists of Kenya. *American Journal of Human Biology* 11(5):658–672.

Pike, M. C., Spicer, D. V., Dahmoush, L., and Press, M. F. 1993. Estrogens, progesterones, normal breast cell proliferation, and breast cancer risk. *Epidemiologic Reviews* 15:17–35.

Pokras, R., and Hufnagel, V. G. 1988. Hysterectomy in the United States, 1965–1984. *American Journal of Public Health* 78(7):852–853.

Pollard, I. 1994. *A Guide to Reproduction: Social Issues and Human Concerns.* New York: Cambridge University Press.

Pollard, T. M., and Hyatt, S. B. 1999. *Sex, Gender, and Health.* New York: Cambridge University Press.

Pouilles, J. M., Tremollieres, F., and Ribot, C. 1993. The effects of menopause on longitudinal bone loss from the spine. *Calcified Tissue International* 52:340–343.

Prado Martínez, C., and Cantó Ferreira, M. 1999. Climaterio en la mujer urbana: aproximación bioantropológica y social sobre su morbilidad. *Anthropología Física Latinoamericana* 2:83–106.

Prebeg, Z., and Bralic, I. 2000. Changes in menarcheal age in girls exposed to war conditions. *American Journal of Human Biology* 12:503–508.

Priestley, C. J., Jones, B. M., Dhar, J., and Godwin, L. 1997. What is normal vaginal flora? *Genitourinary Medicine* 73:23–28.

Profet, M. 1992. Pregnancy sickness as adaptation: a deterrent to maternal ingestion of teratogens. In J. H. Barkow, L. Cosmides, and J. Tooby, eds., *The Adapted Mind: Evolutionary Psychology and the Generation of Culture,* 327–365. New York: Oxford University Press.

Punyahotra, S., Dennerstein, L., and Lehert, P. 1997. Menopausal experiences of Thai women. Part I: Symptoms and their correlates. *Maturitas* 26:1–7.

Purdy, L. 2001. Medicalization, medical necessity, and feminist medicine. *Bioethics* 15(3):248–261.

Rabinowe, S. L., Ravnikar, V. A., Dib, S. A., George, K. L., and Dluhy, R.G. 1989. Premature menopause: monoclonal antibody defined T lymphocyte abnormalities and antiovarian antibodies. *Fertility and Sterility* 51(3):450–454.

Radford, J. A., Lieberman, B. A., Brison, D. R., Smith, A. R., Critchlow, J. D., Russell, S. A., Watson, A. J., Clayton, J. A., Harris, M., Gosden, R. G., and Shalet, S. M. 2001. Orthotopic reimplantation of cryopreserved ovarian cortical strips after high-dose chemotherapy for Hodgkin's lymphoma. *Lancet* 357(9263):1172–1175.

Randhawa, I., Premi, H. K., and Gupta, T. 1987. The age at menopause in women of Himachai Pradesh and the factors affecting the menopause. *Indian Journal of Public Health* 31:40–44.

Randolph, J. F., Jr., Sowers, M., Bondarenko, I. V., Harlow, S. D., Luborsky, J. L., and Little, R. J. 2004. Change in estradiol and follicle-stimulating hormone across the early menopausal transition: effects of ethnicity and age. *Journal of Clinical Endocrinology and Metabolism* 89(4):1555–1561.

Rannevik, G., Jeppsson, S., Johnell, O., Bjerre, B., Laurell-Borulf, Y., and Svanberg, L. 1995. A longitudinal study of the perimenopausal transition: altered profiles of steroid and pituitary hormones, SHBG, and bone mineral density. *Maturitas* 21:103–113.

Raskin, B. 1987. *Hot Flashes: The Novel.* New York: St. Martin's Press.

Reame, N. E., Kelche, R. P., Beitins, I. Z., Yu, M. Y., Zawacki, C. M., and Padmanabhan, V. 1996. Age effects of FSH and pulsatile LH secretion across the menstrual cycle of premenopausal women. *Journal of Clinical Endocrinology and Metabolism* 81:1512–1518.

Rebar, R. W. 2000. Premature ovarian failure. In R. A. Lobo, J. Kelsey, and R. Marcus, eds., *Menopause: Biology and Pathology,* 135–146. New York: Academic Press.

Rebar, R. W., and Connolly, H. V. 1990. Clinical features of young women with hyper-gonadotropic amenorrhea. *Fertility and Sterility* 53:804–810.

Rebato, E. 1988. Ages at menarche and menopause in Basque women. *Collegium Anthropologicum* 12:147–149.

Regalado, A. 2004. Baby is delivered of ovarian tissue previously frozen. *Wall Street Journal,* Sept. 24:B3.

Reichman, B. S., and Green, K. B. 1994. Breast cancer in young women: effect of chemotherapy on ovarian function, fertility, and birth defects. *Journal of the National Cancer Institute Monographs* 16:125–129.

Relethford, J. H. 1997. Hemispheric difference in human skin color. *American Journal of Physical Anthropology* 104:449–457.

———. 2003. *Reflections of Our Past: How Human History Is Revealed in Our Genes.* Boulder, Westview Press.

———. 2005. *The Human Species: An Introduction to Biological Anthropology.* New York: McGraw-Hill.

Revel, A., and Laufer, N. 2002. Protecting female fertility from cancer therapy. *Molecular and Cellular Endocrinology* 187(1–2):83–91.

Reyes Cañizales, A. J., Jackson B., L.A., Ugarte, R., and Gallardo P., J.L. 2005. Ecosensibilidad del climaterio: una aproximación al estudio de la edad en la menopausia en un grupo de mujeres Venezolanas [abstract]. XIII Coloquio Internacional de Antropología Física Juan Comas. Campeche, Mexico, Nov. 6–11.

Reynaud, K., Cortvrindt, R., Verlinde, F., De Schepper, J., Bourgain, C., and Smitz, J. 2004. Number of ovarian follicles in human fetuses with the 45,X karyotype. *Fertility and Sterility* 81:1112–1119.

Reynolds, H. B. 1978. *"To Keep the Tali Strong": Women's Rituals in Tamilnad, India.* Ph.D. diss., University of Wisconsin, Madison.

Reynolds, R. F., and Obermeyer, C. M. 2005. Age at natural menopause in Spain and the United States: results from the DAMES project. *American Journal of Human Biology* 17(3):331–340.

Richardson, S. J., and Nelson, J. F. 1990. Follicular depletion during the menopausal transition. *Annals of the New York Academy of Sciences* 592:13–20.

Richardson, S. J., Senika, V., and Nelson, J. 1987. Follicular depletion during the menopausal transition: evidence for accelerated loss and ultimate exhaustion. *Journal of Clinical Endocrinology and Metabolism* 65(5):1231–1237.

Riessman, C. K. 1983. Women and medicalization: a new perspective. *Social Policy* 14(1):3–18.

Riley, M. W. 1979. Introduction: life-course perspectives. In M. W. Riley, ed., *Aging from Birth to Death: Interdisciplinary Perspectives,* 3–13. Boulder: Westview Press.

———. 1982. Aging and social change. In M. W. Riley, R. P. Abeles, and M. S. Teitelbaum, eds., *Aging from Birth to Death,* vol. 2: *Sociotemporal Perspectives,* 11–26. Boulder: Westview Press.

———. 1986. Overview and highlights of a sociological perspective. In A. Sorensen, F. Weinert, and L. Sherrod, eds., *Human Development and the Life Course: Multidisciplinary Perspectives,* 153–175. Hillsdale, NJ: Lawrence Erlbaum Associates.

Riley, M. W., Abeles, R. P., and Teitelbaum, M. S., eds. 1982. *Aging from Birth to Death,* vol. 2: *Sociotemporal Perspectives.* Boulder: Westview Press.

Rizk, D.E.E., Bener, A., Ezimokhai, M., Hassan, M. Y., and Micallef, R. 1998. The age and symptomatology of natural menopause among United Arab Emirates women. *Maturitas* 29:197–202.

Roberts, C. G., and O'Neill, C. 1995. Increase in the rate of diploidy with maternal age in unfertilized in-vitro fertilization oocytes. *Human Reproduction* 10:2139–2141.

Robinson, W. J. 1938. *Woman: Her Sex and Love Life.* New York: Eugenics Publishing.

Rodstrom, K., Bengtsson, C., Milsom, I., Lissner, L., Sundh, V., and Bjourkelund, C. 2003. Evidence for a secular trend in menopausal age: a population study of women in Gothenburg. *Menopause* 10(6):538–543.

Rodstrom, K., Bengtsson, C., Lissner, L., and Bjourkelund, C. 2005. Reproducibility of self-reported menopause age at the 24-year follow-up of a population study of women in Goteborg, Sweden. *Menopause* 12(3):275–280.

Rogers, A. R. 1993. Why menopause? *Evolutionary Ecology* 7:406–420.

Rosenthal, S. H. 1974. Involutional depression. In S. Arieti, and E. B. Brody, eds., *American Handbook of Psychiatry.* 2nd ed., vol. 3, 694–709. New York: Basic Books.

Rothfield, P. 1997. Menopausal embodiment. In P. A. Komesaroff, P. Rothfield, and J. Daly, eds., *Reinterpreting Menopause: Cultural and Philosophical Issues,* 32–53. New York: Routledge.

Rozenberg, S. C., Fellemans, C., Kroll, M., and Vandromme, J. 2000. The menopause in Europe. *International Journal of Fertility and Women's Medicine* 45:182–189.

Rueda Martinez de Santos, J. R. 1997. Medicalization of menopause and public health. *Journal of Psychosomatic Obstetrics and Gynecology* 18:175–180.

Rulin, M. C., Davidson, A. R., Philliber, S. G., Graves, W. L., and Cushman, L. F. 1993. Long-term effect of tubal sterilization on menstrual indices and pelvic pain. *Obstetrics and Gynecology* 82(1):118–121.

Sacher, G. A. 1978. Evolution of longevity and survival characteristics in mammals. In E. L. Schneider, ed., *The Genetics of Aging,* 151–168. New York: Plenum Press.

Santoro, N. 1996. Hormonal changes in the perimenopause. *Clinical Consultations in Obstetrics and Gynecology* 8:2–8.

Santow, G. 1994. Re: "Long-term risk of hysterectomy among 80,007 sterilized and comparison women at Kaiser Permanente, 1971–1987" [letter]. *American Journal of Epidemiology* 140(7):661.

———. 1995. Education and hysterectomy. *Stockholm Research Reports in Demography,* no. 89. Stockholms Universitet, Stockholm.

Santow, G., and Bracher, M. 1992. Correlates of hysterectomy in Australia. *Social Science and Medicine* 34(8):929–942.

Sarin, A. R., Singla, P., and Sudershan, K. G. 1985. A 5-year clinico-pathological study of 2000 postmenopausal women from northern India. *Asia-Oceania Journal of Obstetrics and Gynaecology* 11:539–544.

Sarrel, L., and Sarrel, P. M. 1994. Helping women decide about hormone replacement therapy: approaches to counseling and medical practices. In G. Berg, and M. Hammar, eds., *The Modern Management of the Menopause: A Perspective for the Twenty First Century,* 499–509. New York: Parthenon Publishing.

Sauer, M. V., Paulson, R. J., and Lobo, R. A. 1992. Reversing the natural decline in human fertility: an extended clinical trial of oocyte donation to women of advanced reproductive age. *Journal of the American Medical Association* 268:1275–1279.

———. 1993. Pregnancy after age 50: application of oocyte donation to women after natural menopause. *Lancet* 341(8841):321–323.

———. 1995. Pregnancy in women 50 or more years of age: outcomes of 22 consecutively established pregnancies from oocyte donation. *Fertility and Sterility* 64(1):111–115.

Scarf, M. 1980. *Unfinished Business: Pressure Points in the Lives of Women.* Garden City, NJ: Doubleday and Company.

Scheffer, G. J., Broekmans, F.J.M., Dorland, M., Habbema, J.D.F., Looman, C.W.N., and te Velde, E. R. 1999. Antral follicle counts by transvaginal ultrasonography are related to age in women with proven natural fertility. *Fertility and Sterility* 72:845–851.

Schilsky, R. L., Sherins, R. J., Hubbard, S. M., Wesley, M. N., Young, R. C., and DeVita, V. T. 1981. Long-term follow up of ovarian function in women treated with MOPP chemotherapy for Hodgkin's disease. *American Journal of Medicine* 71:552–556

Schimmer, A. D., Quartermain, M., Imrie, K., Ali, V., McCrae, J., Stewart, A. K., Crump, M., Derzko, C., and Keating, A. 1998. Ovarian function after autologous bone marrow transplantation. *Journal of Clinical Oncology* 16(7):2359–2363.

Schmidt-Sarosi, C. 1998. Infertility in the older woman. *Clinical Obstetrics and Gynecology* 41(4):940–950.

Schnatz, P. T. 1985. Neuroendocrinology and the ovulation cycle—advances and review. *Advances in Psychosomatic Medicine* 12:4–24.

Scholl, T. O., Hediger, M. L., and Schall, J. I. 1996. Excessive gestational weight gain and chronic disease risk. *American Journal of Human Biology* 8:735–741.

Schwingl, P. J., Hulka, B. S., and Harlow, S. 1994. Risk factors for menopausal hot flashes. *Obstetrics and Gynecology* 84:20–34.

Seifer, D. B., Lambert-Messerlian, G., Hogan, J. W., Gardiner, A. C., Blazar, A. S., and Berk, C. A. 1997. Day 3 serum inhibin-B is predictive of assisted reproductive technologies outcome. *Fertility and Sterility* 67(1):110–114.

Sherman, B. M. 1987. Endocrinologic and menstrual alterations. In D. R. Mishell, ed., *Menopause: Physiology and Pharmacology,* 41–51. Chicago: Year Book Medical.

Sherwin, B. B. 1991. The impact of different doses of estrogen and progestin on mood and sexual behavior in postmenopausal women. *Journal of Clinical Endocrinology and Metabolism.* 72:336–343.

Shinberg, D. S. 1998. An event history analysis of age at last menstrual period: correlates of natural and surgical menopause among midlife Wisconsin women. *Social Science and Medicine* 46(10):1381–1396.

Shumaker, S. A., Legault, C., Thal, L., et al., for the WHIMS Investigators. 2003. Estrogen plus progestin and the incidence of dementia and mild cognitive impairment in postmenopausal women: the Women's Health Initiative Memory Study: a randomized controlled trial. *Journal of the American Medical Association* 289:2651–2662.

Sievert, L. L. 2001a. Aging and reproductive senescence. In P. Ellison, ed., *Reproductive Ecology and Human Evolution,* 267–292. Hawthorne, NY: Aldine de Gruyter.

———. 2001b. Menopause as a measure of population health. *American Journal of Human Biology* 13:429–433.

———. 2003. The medicalization of female fertility: points of significance for the study of menopause. *Collegium Anthropologicum* 27(1):67–78.

Sievert, L. L., and Espinosa-Hernández, G. 2003. Attitudes toward menopause in relation to symptom experience in Puebla, Mexico. *Women and Health* 38(2):93–106.

Sievert, L. L., and Flanagan, E. K. 2005. Geographical distribution of hot flash frequencies: considering climatic influences. *American Journal of Physical Anthropology* 128:437–443.

Sievert, L. L., Freedman, R. R., Zarain García, J., Foster, J. L., Romano, M. C., Longcope, C., and Franz, C. 2002. Measurement of hot flashes by sternal skin conductance and subjective hot flash report in Puebla, Mexico. *Menopause* 9(5):367–376.

Sievert, L. L., González, M. C., and Gómez, M. D. 2004. Factors associated with hot flashes in Asunción, Paraguay [abstract]. *Menopause* 11(6):684.

Sievert, L. L., and Goode-Null, S. K. 2005. Musculoskeletal pain among women of menopausal age in Puebla, Mexico. *Journal of Cross-Cultural Gerontology* 20:127–140.

Sievert, L. L., and Hautaniemi, S. I. 2003. Age at menopause in Puebla, Mexico. *Human Biology* 75(2):205–226.

Sievert, L. L., Obermeyer, C. M., and Price, K. 2006. Determinants of hot flashes and night sweats. *Annals of Human Biology* 33(1):4–16.

Sievert, L. L., Vidovič, M., Horak, H., and Abel, M. 2004. Age and symptom experience at menopause in the Selška Valley, Slovenia. *Menopause* 11(2):223–227.

Sievert, L. L., Waddle, D., and Canali, K. 2001. Marital status and age at natural menopause: considering pheromonal influence. *American Journal of Human Biology* 13:479–485.

Silverman, P. 1987. Introduction: the life course perspective. In P. Silverman, ed., *The Elderly as Modern Pioneers*, 1–16. Indianapolis: Indiana University Press.

Simon, D., Adams, A. M., and Madhavan, S. 2002. Women's social power, child nutrition, and poverty in Mali. *Journal of Biosocial Science* 34:193–213.

Simoons, F. J. 1978. The geographic hypothesis and lactose malabsorption. *American Journal of Digestive Diseases* 23:963–980.

Skarsgard, C., Bjors, E., Nedstrand, E., Wyon, Y., and Hammar, M. 1996. Do women's premenstrual symptoms and their mother's climacteric history predispose them to their own vasomotor symptoms? *Menopause* 3:133–139.

Smith, A.M.A., Dennerstein, L., Morse, C. A., Hopper, J. L., and Green, A. 1992. Costs and benefits of use of commercial market research approaches in large scale surveys. *Medical Journal of Australia* 157(7):504.

Smith, B. H. 1991. Dental development and the evolution of life history in Hominidae. *American Journal of Physical Anthropology* 86:157–174.

Smith, C. G., Almirez, R. G., Berenberg, J., and Asch, R. H. 1983. Tolerance develops to the disruptive effects of Δ^9-tetrahydrocannabinol on primate menstrual cycle. *Science* 219:1453–1455.

Smith, C. G., Besch, N. F., Smith, R. G., and Besch, P. K. 1979. Effect of tetrahydrocannabinol on the hypothalamic-pituitary axis in the ovariectomized rhesus monkey. *Fertility and Sterility* 31: 335–339.

Smith, G. A., and Thomas, R. B. 1998. What could be: biocultural anthropology for the next generation. In A. H. Goodman, and T. L. Leatherman, eds., *Building a New Biocultural Synthesis*, 451–473. Ann Arbor: University of Michigan Press.

Snieder, H., MacGregor, A. J., and Spector, T. D. 1998. Genes control the cessation of a woman's reproductive life: a twin study of hysterectomy and age at menopause. *Journal of Clinical Endocrinology and Metabolism* 83:1875–1880.

Snowdon, D. A. 1990. Early menopause and the duration of postmenopausal life: findings from a mathematical model of life expectancy. *Journal of the American Geriatrics Society* 38(4):402–408.

Snowdon, D. A., Kane, R. L., Beeson, W. L., Burke, G. L., Sprafka, J. M., Potter, J., Hiroyasu, I., Jacobs, D. R., and Phillips, R. L. 1989. Is early natural menopause a biologic marker of health and aging? *American Journal of Public Health* 79:709–714.

Sommer, B., Avis, N., Meyer, P., Ory, M., Madden, T., Kagawa-Singer, M., Mouton, C., Rasor, M. O., and Adler, S. 1999. Attitudes toward menopause and aging across ethnic/racial groups. *Psychosomatic Medicine* 61(6):868–875.

Sonmezer, M., and Oktay, K. 2004. Fertility preservation in female patients. *Human Reproduction Update* 10(3):251–266.

Sorensen, A., Weinert, F., and Sherrod, L. 1986. *Human Development and the Life Course: Multidisciplinary Perspectives.* Hillsdale, NJ: Lawrence Erlbaum Associates.

Soules, M. R., Parrott, E., Rebar, R., Santoro, N., Sherman, S., Utian, W., and Woods, N. F. 2002. Reply to the letter to the editor. *Menopause* 9(6):464–465.

Soules, M. R., Sherman, S., Parrott, E., Rebar, R., Santoro, N., and Utian, W. 2001. Executive summary: States of Reproductive Aging Workshop (STRAW), Park City, Utah, July, 2001. *Menopause* 8(6):402–406.

Sowers, M. F., Crawford, S. L., Sternfeld, B., Morganstein, D., Gold, E. B., Breendale, G. A., Evans, D., Neer, R., Matthews, K., Sherman, S., Lo, A., Weiss, G., and Kelsey, J. 2000. SWAN: A multicenter, multiethnic, community-based cohort study of women and the menopause transition. In R. A. Lobo, J. Kelsey, and R. Marcus, eds., *Menopause: Biology and Pathology,* 175–188. New York: Academic Press.

Sowers, M. R., and La Pietra, M. T. 1995. Menopause: its epidemiology and potential association with chronic diseases. *Epidemiologic Reviews* 17:287–302.

Spence, A. P. 1989. *Biology of Human Aging.* Englewood Cliffs, NJ: Prentice Hall.

Speroff, L., Glass, R. H., and Kase, N. G. 1999. *Clinical Gynecologic Endocrinology and Infertility.* 6th ed. Baltimore: Lippincott Williams and Wilkins.

Spinelli M. G. 2000. Effects of steroids on mood/depression. In R. A. Lobo, J. Kelsey, and R. Marcus, eds., *Menopause: Biology and Pathobiology,* 563–582. New York: Academic Press.

Stanford, J. L., Hartge, P., Brinton, L. A., Hoover, R. N., and Brookmeyer, R. 1987. Factors influencing the age at natural menopause. *Journal of Chronic Diseases* 40:995–1002.

Staropoli, C. A., Flaws, J. A., Bush, T. L., and Moulton, A. W. 1998. Predictors of menopausal hot flashes. *Journal of Women's Health* 7(9):1149–1155.

Stein, K. D., Jacobsen, P. B., Hann, D. M., Greenberg, H., and Lyman, G. 2000. Impact of hot flashes on quality of life among postmenopausal women being treated for breast cancer. *Journal of Pain and Symptom Management* 19(6):436–445.

Stein, Z. A. 1985. A woman's age: childbearing and child rearing. *American Journal of Epidemiology* 121(3):327–342.

Stergachis, A., Shy, K. K., Grothaus, L. C., Wagner, E. H., Hecht, J. A., Anderson, G., Normand, E. H., and Raboud, J. 1990. Tubal sterilization and the long-term risk of hysterectomy. *Journal of the American Medical Association* 264:2893–2898.

Sternfeld, B., Quesenberry, C. P., and Husson, G. 1999. Habitual physical activity and menopausal symptoms: a case-control study. *Journal of Womens Health* 8(1):115–123.

Stevenson, J. C., Crook, D., and Godsland, I. F. 1993. Influence of age and menopause on serum lipids and lipoproteins in healthy women. *Atherosclerosis* 98:83–90.

Stewart, D. E., and Boydell, K. M. 1993. Psychologic distress during menopause: associations across the reproductive life cycle. *International Journal of Psychiatry in Medicine* 23(2):157–162.

Strassman, B. I. 1996. The evolution of endometrial cycles and menstruation. *Quarterly Review of Biology* 71:181–220.

Stroup-Benham, C. A., and Trevino, F. M. 1991. Reproductive characteristics of Mexican-American, mainland Puerto Rican, and Cuban-American women. Data from the Hispanic Health and Nutrition Examination Survey. *Journal of the American Medical Association* 265(2):222–226.

Stuart-Macadam, P. 1995. Breastfeeding in prehistory. In P. Stuart-Macadam, and K. A. Dettwyler, eds., *Breastfeeding: Biocultural Perspectives,* 75–99. Hawthorne, NY: Aldine de Gruyter.

Sukwatana, P., Meekhangvan, J., Tamrongterakul, T., Tanapat, Y., Asavarait, S., and Boonjitrpimon, P. 1991. Menopausal symptoms among Thai women in Bangkok. *Maturitas* 13:217–228.

Swartzman, L. C., Edelberg, R., and Kemmann, E. 1990. The menopausal hot flush: symptom reports and concomitant physiological changes. *Journal of Behavioral Medicine* 13(1):15–30.

Sztein, J., Sweet, H., Farley, J., and Mobraaten, L. 1998. Cryopreservation and orthotopic transplantation of mouse ovaries: new approach in gamete banking. *Biology of Reproduction* 58(4):1071–1074.

Takahata, Y., Koyama, N., and Suzuki, S. 1995. Do the old aged females experience a long post-reproductive life span?: the cases of Japanese macaques and chimpanzees. *Primates* 36(2):169–180.

Tepper, R., Pardo, J., Ovadia, J., and Beyth, Y. 1992. Menopausal hot flushes, plasma calcitonin, and beta-endorphin: A preliminary report. *Gynecologic and Obstetric Investigation* 33(2):98–101.

Tepperman, J., and Tepperman, H. M. 1987. *Metabolic and Endocrine Physiology.* Chicago: Year Book Medical Publishers.

Terwiel, B. J. 1975. *Monks and Magic: An Analysis of Religious Ceremonies in Central Thailand.* Monograph 24, Scandinavian Institute of Asian Studies. London: Curzon Press.

Thomas, R. B., Gage, T. B., and Little, M. A. 1989. Reflections on adaptive and ecological models. In L. A. Little and J. D. Haas, eds., *Human Population Biology: A Transdisciplinary Science,* 296–319. New York: Oxford University Press.

Thomas, F., François, R., Benefice, E., de Meeus, T., and Guegan, J.-F. 2001. International variability of ages at menarche and menopause. *Human Biology* 73(2):271–290.

Thomford, P. J., Jelovsek, F. R., and Mattison, D. R. 1987. Effect of oocyte number and rate of atresia on the age of menopause. *Reproductive Toxicology* 1:41–51.

Thompson, B., Hart, S. A., and Durno, D. 1973. Menopausal age and symptomatology in a general practice. *Journal of Biosocial Science* 5:71–82.

Tilt, E. J. 1882. *The Change of Life, in Health and Disease. A Clinical Treatise on the Diseases of the Ganglionic Nervous System Incidental to Women at the Decline of Life.* 4th ed. Philadelphia: P. Blakiston, Son & Co.

Torgerson, D. J., Avenell, A., Russell, I. T., and Reid, D. M. 1994. Factors associated with age at menopause in women aged 45–49. *Maturitas* 19:83–92.

Torgerson, D. J., Thomas, R. E., Campbell, M. K., and Reid, D. M. 1997. Alcohol consumption and age of maternal menopause are associated with menopause onset. *Maturitas* 26:21–25.

Treloar, A. E. 1974. Menarche, menopause, and intervening fecundability. *Human Biology* 46(1):89–107.

———. 1981. Menstrual cyclicity and the pre-menopause. *Maturitas* 3(3–4):249–64.

Treloar, A. E., Boynton, R. E., Behn, B. G., and Brown, B. W. 1967. Variation of the human menstrual cycle through reproductive life. *International Journal of Fertility* 12(1, pt. 2):77–126.

Treloar, S. A., Do, K.-A., and Martin, N. G. 1998. Genetic influences on the age at menopause. *Lancet* 352:1084–1085.

Treloar, S. A., Sadrzadeh, S., Do, K. A., Martin, N. G., and Lambalk, C. B. 2000. Birth weight and age at menopause in Australian female twin pairs: exploration of the fetal origin hypothesis. *Human Reproduction* 15:55–59.

Trevathan, W. R., Smith, E. O., and McKenna, J. J. 1999. *Evolutionary Medicine*. New York: Oxford University Press.

Turke, P. W. 1988. Helpers at the nest: childcare networks on Ifaluk. In L. Betzig, M. B. Mulder, and P. Turke, eds., *Human Reproductive Behavior: A Darwinian Perspective*, 173–188. New York: Cambridge University Press.

Uphold, C. R., and Susman, E. 1981. Self-reported climacteric symptoms as a function of the relationships between marital adjustment and childrearing stage. *Nursing Research* 30(2):84–88.

Utian, W. H. 1978. Application of cost-effectiveness analysis to post-menopausal estrogen therapy. *Frontiers of Hormone Research* 5:26–39.

———. 1997. What's in a name? [editorial]. *Menopause Management* 6:8.

———. 2001. Semantics, menopause-related terminology, and the STRAW reproductive aging staging system. *Menopause* 8(6):398–401.

van Noord, P.A.H., Dubas, J. S., Dorland, M., Boersma, H., and te Velde, E. 1997. Age at natural menopause in a population-based screening cohort: the role of menarche, fecundity, and lifestyle factors. *Fertility and Sterility* 68(1):95–102.

van Noord, P.A.H., and Kaaks, R. 1991. The effect of wartime conditions and the 1944–45 "Dutch Famine" on recalled menarcheal age in participants of the DOM breast cancer screening project. *Annals of Human Biology* 18:57–70.

van Noord-Zaadstra, B. M., Looman, C. W., Alsbach, H., Habbema, J. D., te Velde E. R., and Karbaat, J. 1991. Delaying childbearing: effect of age on fecundity and outcome of pregnancy. *British Medical Journal* 302(6789):1361–1365.

van Rooij, I. A., Broekmans, F. J., te Velde, E. R., Fauser, B. C., Bancsi, L. F., de Jong, F. H., and Themmen, A. P. 2002. Serum anti-Müllerian hormone levels: a novel measure of ovarian reserve. *Human Reproduction* 17(12):3065–3071.

Varea, C., Bernis, C., Montero, P., Arias, S., Barroso, A., and Gonzalez, B. 2000. Secular trend and intrapopulational variation in age at menopause in Spanish women. *Journal of Biosocial Science* 32:383–393.

Vatuk, S. 1975. The aging woman in India: self-perceptions and changing roles. In A. de Souza, ed., *Women in Contemporary India: Traditional Images and Changing Roles*, 142–163. New Delhi: Manohar.

Velasco, E., Malacara, J. M., Cervantes, F., de Leon, J. D., Davalos, G., and Castillo, J. 1990. Gonadotropins and prolactin serum levels during the perimenopausal period: correlation with diverse factors. *Fertility and Sterility* 53(1):56–60.

Verweij, M. 1999. Medicalization as a moral problem for preventative medicine. *Bioethics* 13(2):89–113.

Vikram, N. K., Pandey, R. M., Misra, A., Sharma, R., Devi, J. R., and Khanna, N. 2003. Non-obese (body mass index <25 kg/m^2) Asian Indians with normal waist circumference have high cardiovascular risk. *Nutrition* 19(6):503–509.

Voda, A. M. 1997. *Menopause, Me, and You: The Sound of Women Pausing*. New York: Harrington Park Press.

Voland, E., and Beise, J. 2002. Opposite effects of maternal and paternal grandmothers on infant survival in historical Krummhörn. *Behavioral Ecology and Sociobiology* 52:435–443.

von Mühlen, D. G., Kritz-Silverstein, D., and Barrett-Conner, E. 1995. A community-based study of menopause symptoms and estrogen replacement in older women. *Maturitas* 22:71–78.

von Mühlen, D., Morton, D., Von Mühlen, C. A., and Barrett-Connor, E. 2002. Postmenopausal estrogen and increased risk of clinical osteoarthritis at the hip, hand, and knee in older women. *Journal of Women's Health and Gender-Based Medicine* 11(6):511–518.

Vuorma, S., Teperi, J., Hurskainen, R., Keskimaki, I., and Kujansuu, E. 1998. Hysterectomy trends in Finland in 1987–1995—a register based analysis. *Acta Obstetricia et Gynecologica Scandinavica* 77(7):770–776.

Wadsworth, M.E.J. 1991. *The Imprint of Time: Childhood, History and Adult Life*. Oxford: Oxford University Press.

Wagner, P. J., Kuhn, S., Petry, L. J., and Talbert, F. S. 1995. Age differences in attitudes toward menopause and estrogen replacement therapy. *Women and Health* 23(4):1–16.

Walker, M. L. 1995. Menopause in female rhesus monkeys. *American Journal of Primatology* 35:59–71.

Wallace, W. H., and Kelsey, T. W. 2004. Ovarian reserve and reproductive age may be determined from measurement of ovarian volume. *Human Reproduction* 19(7):1612–1617.

Wassertheil-Smoller, S., Hendrix, S. L., Limacher, M., et al., for the WHI Investigators. 2003. Effect of estrogen plus progestin on stroke in postmenopausal women: the Women's Health Initiative: a randomized trial. *Journal of the American Medical Association* 289:2673–2684.

Wasti, S., Robinson, S. C., Akhtar, T., Khan, S., and Badaruddin, N. 1993. Characteristics of menopause in three socioeconomic urban groups in Karachi, Pakistan. *Maturitas* 16:61–69.

Weir, B. J., and Rowlands, I. W. 1977. Ovulation and atresia. In L. Zuckerman, and B. J. Weir, eds., *The Ovary*, 265–301. New York: Academic.

Weissman, M. M. 1979. The myth of involutional melancholia. *Journal of the American Medical Association* 242(8):742–744.

Weissman, M. M., and Olfson, M. 1995. Depression in women: implications for health care research. *Science* 269:799–801.

Weller, A. 1998. Human pheromones: communication through body odour. *Nature* 392:126–127.

Whelan, E. A., Sandler, D. P., McConnaughey, D. R., and Weinberg, C. R. 1990. Menstrual and reproductive characteristics and age at natural menopause. *American Journal of Epidemiology* 131:625–632.

White, C. 2002. Second long term HRT trial stopped early. *British Medical Journal* 325:987.

Whitehead, M. 1994. The Pieter van Keep memorial lecture. In G. Berg, and M. Hammar, eds., *The Modern Management of the Menopause: A Perspective for the Twenty First Century*, 1–13. New York: Parthenon Publishing.

Whitehead, M. I., Whitcroft, S.I.J., and Hillard, T. C. 1993. *An Atlas of the Menopause*. New York: Parthenon.

Wilbur, J., Miller, A. M., Montgomery, A., and Chandler, P. 1998. Sociodemographic characteristics, biological factors, and symptom reporting in midlife women. *Menopause* 5(1):43–51.

Wiley, A. 1992. Adaptation and the biocultural paradigm in medical anthropology: a critical review. *Medical Anthropology Quarterly* 6:216–236.

———. 2004. *An Ecology of High-Altitude Infancy: A Biocultural Perspective.* New York: Cambridge University Press.

Williams, G. C. 1957. Pleiotropy, natural selection, and the evolution of senescence. *Evolution* 11:398–411.

Wilson, R. A. 1966. *Feminine Forever.* New York: Evans.

Wise, P. M., Kashon, M. L., Krajnak, K. M., Rosewell, K. L., Cai, A., Scarbrough, K., Harney, J. P., McShane, T., Lloyd, J. M., and Weiland, N. G. 1997. Aging of the female reproductive system: a window into brain aging. *Recent Progress in Hormone Research* 52:279–305.

Wood, J. W. 1994. *Dynamics of Human Reproduction: Biology, Biometry, Demography.* New York: Aldine de Gruyter.

Wood, J. W., Holman, D. J., and O'Connor, K. A. 2001. Did menopause evolve by antagonistic pleiotropy? In *Homo unsere Herkunft und Zukunft,* Proceedings 4. Kongress der Gesellschaft für Anthropologie (GfA), 483–490. Göttingen: Cuvillier Verlag.

Wood, J. W., Johnson, P. L., and Campbell, K. L. 1985. Demographic and endocrinological aspects of low natural fertility in highland New Guinea. *Journal of Biosocial Science* 17:57–79.

Wood, J. W., Weeks, S. C., Bentley, G. R., and Weiss, K. M. 1994. Human population biology and the evolution of aging. In D. Crews, and R. Garruto, eds., *Biological Anthropology and Aging: Perspectives on Human Variation over the Life Span,* 19–75. New York: Oxford University Press.

Woods, N. F., Falk, S., Saver, B., Stevens, N., Taylor, T., Moreno, R., and MacLaren, A. 1997. Deciding about using hormone therapy for prevention of diseases of advanced age. *Menopause* 4(2):105–114.

Woods, N. F., and Mitchell, E. S. 1999. Anticipating menopause: observations from the Seattle Midlife Women's Health Study. *Menopause* 6(2):167–173.

Woods, N. F., Mitchell, E. S., and Mariella, A. 2003. Observations from the Seattle Midlife Women's Health Study [abstract]. Fifteenth Biennial Conference of the Society for Menstrual Cycle Research, June 5–7.

Worcester, N., and Whatley, M. H. 1992. The selling of HRT: playing on the fear factor. *Feminist Review* 41:1–26.

World Health Organization (WHO). 1981. *Research on the Menopause.* WHO Technical Report Series no. 670. Geneva: World Health Organization.

———. 1995. *Physical Status: The Use and Interpretation of Anthropometry.* Geneva: World Health Organization.

———. 1996. *Research on the Menopause in the 1990s.* WHO Technical Report Series no. 866. Geneva: World Health Organization.

World Health Organization (WHO)–International Society of Hypertension. 1999. Guidelines for the Management of Hypertension. Guidelines Subcommittee. *Journal of Hypertension* 17:151–183.

Worthman, C. M. 1993. Biocultural interactions in human development. In M. E. Pereira, and L. A. Fairbanks, eds., *Juvenile Primates: Life History, Development, and Behavior,* 339–358. New York: Oxford University Press.

————. 1999. Emotions: you can feel the difference. In A. L. Hinton, ed., *Biocultural Approaches to the Emotions*, 41–74. Cambridge: Cambridge University Press.

Worthman, C. M., and Kohrt, B. 2005. Receding horizons of health: biocultural approaches to public health paradoxes. *Social Science and Medicine* 61(4):861–878.

Worthman, C. M., and Kuzara, J. 2005. Life history and the early origins of health differentials. *American Journal of Human Biology* 17(1):95–112.

Writing Group for the Women's Health Initiative Investigators. 2002. Risks and benefits of estrogen plus progestin in health postmenopausal women: principal results from the Women's Health Initiative randomized controlled trial. *Journal of the American Medical Association* 288(3):321–333.

Wynn, T. 2002. Archaeology and cognitive evolution. *Behavioral and Brain Sciences* 25:389–438.

Wyshak, G. 2004. Menopausal symptoms and psychological distress in women with and without tubal sterilization. *Psychosomatics* 45:403–413.

Zeserson, J. M. 2001. How Japanese women talk about hot flushes: implications for menopause research. *Medical Anthropology Quarterly* 15:189–205.

Zola, I. K. 1972. Medicine as an institution of social control. *Sociological Review* 20(4):487–504.

————. 1983. *Socio-Medical Inquiries: Recollections, Reflections, and Reconsiderations.* Philadelphia: Temple University Press.

INDEX

ABOUT THE AUTHOR

As an undergraduate, Lynnette Leidy Sievert majored in nursing and Spanish at Bloomsburg University in Pennsylvania. She found her first nursing job in Albuquerque, where she discovered biological anthropology, thanks to Henry Harpending and the University of New Mexico. She completed her Ph.D. in biological anthropology at the State University of New York at Albany. Lynnette has been traveling to Mexico since 1979. When not in Puebla, Lynnette lives in Gill, Massachusetts, with her husband and two cats. She is a professor of anthropology at the University of Massachusetts Amherst.